Sleep Your \

Over thirty years ago, **Khurs**
at IIT Bombay, discovered rr
courses. They had both always wanted to make a difference to the people around them, and so, in their early twenties, they chose the unconventional path of being Art of Living teachers. Since then, they have taught Yoga and Meditation to hundreds of thousands of people in more than 35 countries worldwide.

Besides this book, they have co-authored two other books: *Ready, Study, Go! and Happiness Express*. Their first two books have sold more than 100,000 copies and have been translated to Hindi, Tamil and Bulgarian. They are sought-after speakers, and are invited across the world to speak on a variety of topics. They have an award winning YouTube channel **www.youtube.com/bndtv**. Some of their videos on YouTube have more than a million views.

They are Craniosacral Therapists and have created small miracles for people through this powerful alternative healing modality. In 2016, they set up a centre to teach this healing technique. For more about Craniosacral Therapy, visit **www.sstcha.com**.

Khurshed is a registered Bach Flower Therapist, and teaches all three professional certification levels of the Bach Flower Remedy training for the Bach Centre, UK. Navigate to **www.bachflowers.in** for more details.

Dinesh is a fitness enthusiast and enjoys his daily workouts. Khurshed loves nature and long walks. They enjoy reading, music and movies with happy endings. They live amidst nature at Art of Living's picturesque retreat in rural Bangalore.

Praise for the book

When you are curious enough, the answers will find their way to you. My intense curiosity on the subject of sleep has brought me to this book. And finally in a form and style that is lucid. The detailing is incredible. In our caffeine-induced adrenaline pumped lifestyles, we knew sleep could be the perfect antidote but we haven't been using it right. Khurshed and Dinesh reveal a powerful sequence of lifestyle choices that can help us unlock the true potential of sleep.

Sleep has finally been released from the clutches of the 'laziness' tag that it was so unwittingly tied with for generations. This is a book that I would happily take to bed!

— **Harsh Goenka,**
Chairman, RPG Enterprises

A fascinating linkage between Success & Sleep—one almost wonders why the world hasn't taken Sleep more seriously before.

Equally, a powerful framework to revisit your goals—and work toward them more effectively!

— **Bart Janssens**
Senior Partner & Managing Director, Boston Consulting Group

This is so much more than a self-help book about the science of sleep and the importance of good sleep for true success! Khurshed and Dinesh show us how to remove the monsters in our mind—negative self-talk, self-doubt and low self-esteem—to unlock the secret of being successful, and not just achieving success in life.

Sleep Your Way to Success carves out a clear path towards achieving balance, purpose, meaning and fulfilment in life. A must read for those with a growth mindset who want to make positive changes in any sphere of their life.

— **Dr. Rati Godrej MD**

Sleep Your Way to Success is a remarkable powerhouse of a book that helps us to unleash the amazing restorative powers of sleep, and its transformational capacity to impact our ability to succeed.

Masterfully written, with simplicity of purpose and clarity of thought, the authors explain the science of how sleep affects our state of mind, and provide actionable insights to implement and position oneself for success.

Success means different things to different people, particularly at different stages of life. This book guides the reader to discover what success means to them, and shares simple techniques on how to literally sleep their way towards enriching their wakeful lives.

This gem from Bawa and Dinesh, replete with their inimitable wit and wisdom, is an absolute delight to read and an excellent gift that any reader can give themselves!

— **Rajiv Kaul**
Former President, Leela Palaces, Hotels and Resorts

Sleep Your Way to Success is an inspiring, revelatory book, filled with anecdotes, research, self-experimented data, and simple but impactful suggestions to success and well-being—two things that often don't go hand-in-hand.

My favourite chapters? The FAQ on Sleep, The Pizza of life and Adding by Subtracting. These few pages will change the way you look at your life.

— **Kewal Handa**
Former Chairman, Union Bank of India

I had absolutely no idea that something as simple as sleeping could make me feel good, look great, perform better, and be the basis of fantastic relationships. I am pretty sure many people, me included, felt that sleep is a waste of time. This book convinced me that it is not. I particularly loved the fact that the authors have spelt out exactly what needs to be done (or not done) to tap into the awesome power of restful, rejuvenative sleep.

The second part of the book—the chapters revolving around the idea of success take a completely different approach from what is the norm. Instead of telling you what success is, you are encouraged, through a series of exercises to define your own idea of success. Then, go on to create an actionable road map towards it.

Bawa and Dinesh are known for their simple yet profound insights, and effective methodology towards creating solutions for the stickier challenges that life throws at you. *Sleep Your Way to Success* is packed with this wisdom and you will be a better, more effective person through reading it.

— **V.S.S. Mani,**
Founder & CEO, JustDial

I really enjoyed *Sleep Your Way to Success*—simple conversational language, clear messages and takeaways. I have learned so much about sleep and sleep hygiene—I had no idea alarm clocks were health risks, for example. Equally, the success chapters gave me lots of ideas to reprioritise and optimise my day-to-day schedule. Life is easier and more fun after reading this book.

— **Kanchan Samtani**
Senior Partner and Managing Director, Boston Consulting Group

Implementing just one thing from the sleep section of this remarkable book has actually made me look and feel considerably younger! I had deprioritised sleep for decades, always justifying to myself that I was happy and high-functioning. Bawa and Dinesh reframed my thinking on sleep—I have now put aside superhero tactics, and give sleep its due importance.

This book is equally a ticket to success—like you never imagined before. Through their keen understanding of the mind, the authors walk you through a journey of reflection around why you do what you do, and invite you to operate from your 'courage zone'." Several insightful chapters in this book are a 'productivity compass', pointing to little changes that can dramatically boost one's productivity. The most extraordinary shift personally was through their simple, but life-altering '5 ½ half minute' rule.

A most insightful read—one that undoubtedly everyone will benefit from.

— **Nisheeta Bajaj Janssens,**
Global executive coach to CEOs, Author, Advisor (various organisations)

Being a chess player by profession, I am perfectly aware of how critically important it is to stay sharp and relaxed at the same time. Otherwise, you get instantly punished. Mental and physical health are of utmost importance for success, and enough good quality sleep is the vital ingredient to ensure these remain optimal.

Khurshed and Dinesh explain this fact in their typical crystal clear style, full of humour and wisdom. There is a soothing aspect to their writing that always makes me smile and feel good. I truly appreciate the amount of self-experimentation and research that has gone into writing this book.

Their pieces on success are spot-on, and with this book you are truly armed to sleep well, dream big—and figure out a plan to actually make those dreams come true.

— **Surya Shekhar Ganguly**
Chess Grandmaster, Arjuna Award Winner 2005

Having read *Happiness Express* and *Ready Steady Go*, I knew with absolute certainty that Bawa and Dinesh's new book on Sleep would be a treasury of wisdom. And that's exactly what it turned out to be. The book is truly an eye-opener, making us realise the importance of deep sleep for creating magic at a deeper level, thereby healing and energising the body and soul.

It is a must-read for all ages, and is a valuable tool to help us achieve true happiness and success.

— **Navyata Goenka**
Former investment banker & mother of 3

Loved it... the book handles a touchy (at least for me) topic with a sensitive practicality. I was astounded to know of all that could be set right by this most important of renovation functions for our bodies—sleep!

Much has been said, and much has been written in the past about sleep and its benefits. And God knows several of us have been keen consumers of it, but never did any of that stay with so much conviction, as it does after reading *Sleep Your Way to Success*. Simply because, as always—Bawa and Dinesh make it simple, relatable, humorous and surmountable!

The book explores the idea of success, expertly intertwining it with sleep. You will feel an intense eagerness to make a beginning at revamping your schedule to achieve the big goals and dreams of your life.

I would recommend this book across all age groups—it is exactly in line with Bawa and Dinesh's universality!

— **Bhavana Bindra**
MD South Asia, REHAU

Sleep is nature's superpower. Science is unambiguously clear that a good night's sleep positively impacts our well-being, both physically and mentally. This fact is often under-rated and not well understood. *Sleep Your Way to Success* hits this point home and how! The narrative flows smoothly, switching between the logic and science of sleep, to practical suggestions and daily tips that will help you move unerringly towards success.

— **Amit Nayyar,**
Former President, Paytm, ex-Goldman Sachs

The authors urge you to read *Sleep Your Way to Success* one short chapter at a time. I found this to be impossible. Once I started reading, I simply couldn't put it down. I wanted to get it all in one shot. The topics covered are critical to success and well-being, but not talked about enough. The writing style is easy and conversational and many times I felt as if the authors were talking to me and engaging me. I could easily comprehend and internalise even the more technical parts of the book.

Over the last 17 years, I have worked in extremely competitive workplaces and have seen a lot of folks compromise on well-being, as they chase the mirage of success. This book allows you to comprehensively define your own version of success in all its multiple dimensions. It then goes on to showing you the 'Hows' of achieving that success in a healthy balanced way.

It's a great read—almost a manual to define and achieve success in a truly sustainable way.

— **Chanchal Bansal**
Business Leader, Google

An eye opening book on closing the eyes for the best of reasons—Sleep!

This book is a product of research and personal experience—and it shows. Bawa and Dinesh take us through their personal stories of how they discovered and implemented the knowledge of sleeping. I find this book authentic, practical and relatable for anyone living in today's super busy, moving-at-light-speed, crammed world.

The part which talks about sleep and new moms especially struck a chord with me. As a mother of two, along with a full-fledged corporate job and an extremely active community life, sleep would often be a trade-off. Not anymore!

If you are looking for a book to snuggle with, pick this one!

— **Sreekala Sunderrajan,**
Director - People and Culture Programme Management, Gojek

This topic of this incredible book is deeply personal to me. In the year 2008, I fell asleep on the wheel driving at 70 miles per hour with my whole family in the car. In the milliseconds of sleep driving, the car drove off into a grass patch and turned 180 degrees to a full stop. It is truly a miracle that I live to write about the incident today. I first hand discovered the NEED to sleep well. It can literally save your life!

Bawa and Dinesh beautifully present the science and art of a good night sleep. This book can help every individual sleep better, which in my opinion, is a prerequisite to being successful. With the recharge of a good night's sleep, you will be ready to implement the numerous success strategies they share from their life experiences in the book. The genius behind the success strategies is their simplicity—easy to learn and implement, yet profound in its impact.

This is a great book to have by your bedside!

— **Rajneesh Gupta**
Global Vice President, Intuit

SLEEP
YOUR WAY TO
SUCCESS

Khurshed Batliwala & **Dinesh** Ghodke

Illustrations by
Gowrishankar Venkatraman

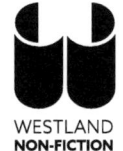

WESTLAND
NON-FICTION

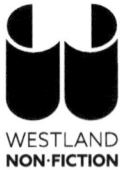

WESTLAND
NON-FICTION

First published by Westland Non-Fiction, an imprint of Westland Publications Private Limited, in 2021

1st Floor, A Block, East Wing, Plot No. 40, SP Infocity, Dr MGR Salai, Perungudi, Kandanchavadi, Chennai 600096

Westland, the Westland logo, Westland Non-Fiction and the Westland Non-Fiction logo are the trademarks of Westland Publications Private Limited, or its affiliates.

Copyright © Khurshed Batliwala and Dinesh Ghodke, 2021

ISBN: 9789391234782

The views and opinions expressed in this work are the authors' own and the facts are as reported by them, and the publisher is in no way liable for the same.

All rights reserved
Book design by New Media Line Creations, New Delhi 110062

No part of this book may be reproduced, or stored in a retrieval system, or transmitted in any form or by any means, electronic, mechanical, photocopying, recording, or otherwise, without express written permission of the publisher.

*Fondly dedicated to Gurudev Sri Sri Ravishankar
—the One who awakens us by making us close our eyes*

Power Sleep Blueprint
A Masterclass

Our mission is to empower 1 million people enhance their sleeping experience, and so, harness the awesome power of Nature's Super Energiser – Sleep.

Science has proved beyond a doubt, that proper sleep makes you younger, healthier and smarter - a combination that propels your success at jet speed, no matter what you do.

We would love to welcome you to our tribe of delighted sleepers.

Visit **www.booksbybnd.com/powersleepblueprint** and register, to watch a masterclass – Power Sleep Blueprint, worth Rs.999/- for FREE, that we have created especially for you.

We hope you enjoy reading our book, as much as we enjoyed writing it for you.

Good Night and Sweet Dreams.

Contents

Preface	XIV
Acknowledgements	XXI
Ode to Sleep by Nadir Godrej	XXV
Foreword by Luke Coutinho	XXVII

Sleep — 1

Why Sleep	3
Three Questions	10
Falling Asleep	15
Sleep and Meditation	33
The Bedroom	39
The Winding Down Ritual	56
The Art of Waking Up	66
Sleep and the Three Vital Energies	78
Babies and Sleep	89
Frequently Asked Questions About Sleep	114

Success — 139

The Monster in Your Head	141
The Pizza of Life	148
Goal Sculpting	158
Superpowers	166
The Expertise Trap	170
Lines	178

Letting Go	186
Adding by Subtracting	192
Dancing with Dopamine	202
Allies and Power-ups	218
Karma and Destiny	231

Appendix — 236

Three Magic Plants for the Bedroom	237
A Shopping Guide	241
Sri Sri Ravi Shankar	251
The Art of Living Foundation Courses	253
Integrated Craniosacral Therapy	261

Workshops with Khurshed and Dinesh — 265

Bach Flower Remedies	266
The Power of Sleep Workshop	270
Study Sutras	272
Mathemagic	274

Bibliography — 276

Preface

The most sophisticated mobile phone in the world will become nothing more than an expensive paperweight if it is not regularly charged. All its features, its apps, its amazing abilities to make stunning photos and videos—all that lavish technology becomes worthless when the battery runs out.

We and our bodies are much the same. We have been created with ultra-sophisticated, fantastically complex organic technology. We can do myriad things. We can cook amazingly tasty food, write beautiful prose and poetry, create music that can lift our spirits or move us to tears, think up things like string theory and quantum physics, make brilliant movies, smile and laugh and cry and experience the most exquisite of emotions—love. We can take care of each other and are capable of immense compassion. We have even managed to go to the moon and beyond.

But just like our phones, we need to regularly recharge ourselves. Otherwise, we become exhausted, dull, angry, frustrated and fearful. We become the antithesis of the glory of being human.

To charge our phones, we use electricity. To charge ourselves, we need to sleep.

Sleep is the most neglected, often completely overlooked way of feeling amazing and looking great. Unfortunately, a vast majority of us consider sleeping to be a waste of time. People all over the world lament: If only I didn't have to sleep so much, I would get so much more done. Understand this: you get things done *because* you sleep. And most people are not getting enough of it.

There are 3 more ways we can recharge ourselves. Through food, through our breath, and by culturing our minds to become serene, calm and happy. There is a lot of literature out there on how to eat healthy. The secrets of the power of the breath can be yours when you practice Pranayama. Yoga and meditation are ancient techniques, excellent for refining the mind. All these are best learned from a qualified teacher.

People with unruffled and cheerful minds can create an explosion of peace around them. They can instantly make you feel at ease as soon as you are with them. These people make you relaxed and in their company, all your tensions melt away. A settled mind brings tremendous feelings of well-being into the environment. And this makes it a formidable source of energy in this day and age. Culturing your mind to become like this is the practice of Meditation. Some might call it Mindfulness. Just like Pranayama, meditation is best learned from a qualified teacher. I would heartily recommend Gurudev Sri Sri Ravi Shankar's Art of Living series of courses that guide you on how to go deep within yourself. More information is sprinkled throughout this book and in the appendix.

While meditation, unlike sleep, requires guidance and training, everyone is born with the ability to rejuvenate themselves through sleep. No guidance required. Yet, huge masses of people across the world suffer from the terrible consequences of sleep deprivation.

Hence, this book.

I have organised this book into short informative pieces about sleep—why one should sleep, what are the benefits of great sleep and the hazards of not getting enough sleep. Included too are tips on inculcating habits that will ensure you are maximising the benefits of your time in bed. The second section of this book explores the idea of success—what you would need to do, or not do, to realise your big life goals.

I would recommend that you read each of these pieces curled up snugly in your bed, just before going to sleep. Or first thing when you awaken in the morning.

Though you might be sorely tempted to, don't read this entire book in one go. Keep this book on your bedside table and read one or two chapters each night. Some chapters may be a little long and you are welcome to read just parts of them each night. The last thoughts we have before we sleep can make a humungous difference to the quality of our sleep and hence to the quality of our lives.

I suffered through a few months of terrible insomnia and know firsthand the debilitating effects of compromised sleep. Ironically, I used all those sleepless nights to research about sleep.

Many pieces in this book are based on this research that I did on the work of many other amazing people. I went through tons of books (some of which are mentioned in the bibliography at the end) and scanned countless websites. I did a lot of experimenting with all that I learned. The result—I cured myself of my insomnia without resorting to any sort of allopathic medication whatsoever. It was a long journey of distilling all that I felt was practical and feasible, and modifying and supplementing it to make it my own. Having said this, I acknowledge that I stand on the shoulders of giants, and I am thankful to them.

Most of us are missing out on the flabbergasting benefits that a good night's sleep can bestow on us. And that's what this book is all about. To borrow a phrase from P.G. Wodehouse—I hope your gast becomes as flabbered as mine when you finish reading this book, implement at least some of what I recommend, and you too start to enjoy the incredible benefits of great sleep. I am pretty sure your gast will be even more flabbered when you get to the second part of the book that talks about success. You will get to define your own version of success. Then you will see how to create an environment geared for success. Finally, you will be able to come up with a strategic action plan that will take you towards the life you dream about.

Here is to your dreams coming true, and a healthier, younger, sexier and smarter you!

Good Night!
Jai Gurudeva!
Bawa n Dinesh

P.S.: The pronouns we and I are used interchangeably in the book—both mean Bawa and Dinesh.

Acknowledgements

We feel grateful and joyous each day as we continue to bask in the ginormous blessings from our beloved Gurudev Sri Sri Ravi Shankar.

Dinesh still is and always will be the solidity of the Himalayas and the love of a few saints, rolled into one. Life is absolutely incredible because of him.

Immense love and gratitude for our parents—they made us who we are.

We are thankful beyond measure …

To Gowrishankar for being there, and for being patient with me as I bounced countless ideas off him. And for the exquisite cover, and all the fun illustrations you will find in this book.

To Dr Ankita Dhelia for her osteopathic treatments. This book couldn't have been possible if she hadn't used her extraordinary skills to keep me fit and healthy despite the long hours of sitting that creating this book required.

To Abhiram and Sunny for the work that you guys so cheerfully do, both online and offline, allowing Dinesh and me the luxury of time.

To Lalit for introducing me to the joy of exercise.

To Nisheeta for all the amazing discussions.

To all the mums who took the time to candidly write out how they coped with their newborn babies and managed to stay more or less sane, even though they were utterly sleep deprived. The Babies and Sleep chapter couldn't have been possible without all of you.

To Devang for his mom-made chikki and chutney and dal … and all the fun and laughter.

To Bhanu Didi for her music, her love and her sweet gentleness with everyone.

To Ajay and Madhu for their encouragement.

To Arvind and Srivi for ensuring we look as great as we feel.

To Dr Unni Nilanjan for taking a LOT of time off and going over the ayurveda aspects of this book. Special thanks to Dr Pinkita and Dr Yogeshwar Chippa for their suggestions and help.

To our old, old Vaidji in Kolkata, Kaviraj ji, for the almost miraculous ayurvedic concoctions that make life that much easier.

To Sakshi, Shiv and Amarja and Raghav for the delicious lunches.

To the ever-helpful Sunit Kaluskar, our go-to person for anything ashram-related.

To Chandu bhai and Deepak, our guys (pun intended) from the ashram Gaushala for all those sumptuous Sunday mornings.

To Shavina for being ever ready to pamper us, even before we know it.

To Sowmya for ensuring that the zoom tech on all our courses worked and for giving her time freely and generously to organise courses for us.

To Poornima V. Ramchand (Shantu) for being the ultra-generous wonderful person she is—and for the lovely conversations.

To Tamanna, Chahat and Prakriti for the treats from the city.

To Manak for guiding us through the stars.

Acknowledgements

To Atin and Pooja for help with marketing … and all the fun!

To Hanoz and Rimpy for their supreme generosity.

To Kapil, Puja and darling Aarna for the good times in London. Looking forward to meeting up in person.

To Swami Vijayanand Saraswati, Govind, Hitesh and team from our exquisite Rishikesh Ashram for going out of their way to make us comfortable during our frequent visits there.

As always, to Prama and late Ranji Bhandari for sharing their beautiful home with us and for the fantastic food and charming stories.

To Alok for sparking my interest in things electrical.

To Lorenzo for creating the last few illustrations in record time, so the book could go into print on schedule.

To Kushal and Alakh for all the support and all the love.

To Shailendra, our house help for taking care of the small things, so we could focus on the big ones.

To Perviz, my sister, and Carl, her husband, for being there, and Aarman, Ahun and Bhuvana, their children, for all the problems and craziness they create.

To Harshal for singing.

To Chirag for continuing to learn … and being a great sport.

To Abhay Joshi for those little and big things that make our lives easier.

To Chaital, Milan and their families for all the lovely times.

To Shobha and Swami for welcoming me to their lovely home in Chennai every time I go there.

To Jai and Pramod Khanna for being great friends.

To Adi Kabra for being our man Friday in Hyderabad. He is actually Monday, Tuesday, Wednesday and Thursday as well. We give him the weekend off.

To all our colleagues—brilliant Art of Living teachers and volunteers on the Inergyworld team—Manisha, Dhara,

Rashmin, Ruchi, Sourav, Ramnik, Amit Mahadik, Himanshu, Sonam and Poonam… thanks!

To everyone on our Craniosacral Therapy team—Lalit, Rima, Sowmya, Sunita, Divya, Swami, Manish, Rimpy, Aruna we could never have run the course without you.

To Dr Rangana Chaudhary for teaching us EFT and NLP and being such a dear friend.

To Braj Mohan Das for the solid training he gave us on our coaching journey.

To Nirmal, Avinash and Mahika for being a part of so many adventures with us.

To all our students—you trusted us to teach you.

To the chefs at Café Vishala—Padmnav, Kuldeep, Prasad and a host of others—who provided us with the much-needed food and drink whenever required.

To Bali, and all the people who accompanied us for the Vigyan Bhairav course there. It was highly rejuvenating and so much fun—I pray that we can start travelling to all these beautiful places again soon.

To Debasri who used to work at Westland for saying 'Yes' … again!

To my editor, Karthik, and the staff at Westland for their support and patience.

A deep gratitude to those who've read bits and pieces, suggested ideas to make this book even better, and generously given advance reviews.

And to you, dear reader, thank you for buying this book and reading it. We hope you will sleep better—and all your dreams come true. Well, not all. Just the nice ones!

Jai Gurudev!
Love,
Bawa n Dinesh

Ode to Sleep
— Nadir Godrej,
Chairman, Godrej Industries

Now Sleep *Your Way to Success*
Does sound risqué, I must confess,
But thoughtful readers surely know
To ignore the innuendo,
And take a very serious look
At this amazingly useful book.

Now lack of sleep can cause a mess,
While proper sleep leads to success.
A fresh recharge is what's required,
So for success you will be wired,
Get the right kind of sleep,
That is both long as well as deep.
You can't perform if you are drowsy …
And with eight hours you won't feel lousy.

All conditions must be right
No loud sounds, or any light.
Before you sleep, you must be calm,
Then, your sleep's a soothing balm.
As every stage has a role,
Good, balanced sleep—this is the goal.

Deep sleep leads to rejuvenation
And dreaming states, to inspiration.
Once inspired and free of stress,
Undoubtedly, you'll taste success.
Brief naps of course, can be an aid …
Yet, they mustn't be overplayed.

Meditate, and you will transcend
Into states you couldn't comprehend.
Now severe stress is very taxing
But meditation is peaceful and relaxing
So, meditation is really very good.
It should be clearly understood,
Just meditating, without sleeping well,
Will make your body and mind rebel.
Towards success, you'll gravitate
If you both sleep and meditate.

Keep all I say well in sight,
But read the book to get it right.
Avoid the trap of sleeping less,
Sleep properly, enjoy success.
Our deepest thanks, Dinesh and Bawa!
Congratulations! Wah! Wah! Wah!

Foreword by Luke Coutinho

Who doesn't want to be successful? But are you focusing on just success or 'true' success that doesn't cost you your health? Does your definition of success include 'health'?

The title of the book may at first sound pretty contradictory to what social media, internet, newspapers and magazines portray. Today, the success of any person is believed to be equal to the number of nights sacrificed. We have been fooled and brainwashed into believing that we need to live a particular way to be successful. We need to compromise on sleep to be a successful employee, a business tycoon, achieve our targets, get good grades, etc. We judge our success based on what it looks like from the exterior—position earned, status earned, money earned, the kind and number of cars owned, handbags and clothes, not realising that all of this means NOTHING without health. Kids today look at social media and stories of billionaires, business tycoons and others who only show the good and flashy side of their lives.

What we see is just their success, not 'behind the scenes', not their blood reports, health, pain, suffering, restlessness, anxiety, sleeping pills popped and drugs taken to maintain this façade because they have abused their bodies. You may think that successful people are happy. Sadly, that is not always the case. Contrary to what's believed, suicides, depression and broken relationships are at their highest amongst them. In fact, when I noticed how top executives and CEOs, despite having it all, suffered from so many lifestyle diseases, obesity, poor emotional health and not being able to enjoy what they built, it served as an ignition point for me to fill this huge gap and inspired me to work in the field of integrative and lifestyle medicine and coach individuals on sleep and its importance.

Sleep is everything and it's a myth that the most successful people sleep less. Sleep rejuvenates, repairs, heals, protects, grows, balances and does so much more. Human beings are the only species that sacrifice 'sleep' to fulfil their career, professional, social and personal goals, to live and achieve more. Burnout due to lack of rest, sleep and focus on health or on eating right is a common phenomenon today. This results in chronic lifestyle diseases, deaths, more unhappiness and a feeling of emptiness, as has been identified by the World Health Organisation (WHO). There are enough instances and scientific evidence to support the connection between sleep deprivation and sickness. It is the number one reason for low immunity, poor growth, delayed healing, bad moods, mood swings, crazy cravings, belly fat and rapid ageing, all of which are reasons why people don't succeed in life.

Sleep is a free drug. I guess that's why it's also taken for granted by the human species. Investing in your sleep is a massive investment in your health and life. In fact, night shift is classified as a 'carcinogen', which means it is cancer-causing, yet we take sleep for granted. Often people in their defence will say, 'But I am resilient.' This is a very careless statement. Building a company, a brand or success of any kind at the cost of health is failure. Not success.

Rest is where magic happens. When we rest, we rest the body, mind and heart. Thinking the faster we move, the faster we will achieve our goals and wealth is a huge misunderstanding. Rest daily as it will rejuvenate every cell in you. You can still achieve what you want, but with adequate rest, you will be able to do so without destroying the beauty of the body, mind and heart.

The science of sleep is undebatable. The laws of nature never change, like the laws of gravity, motion, electricity, cause and effect, no matter how advanced and jetset our lifestyle gets. All of us need to understand that each of us has a set point, a threshold, beyond which our bodies will crash. Abuse your body how much ever you want to, but there will be a point when it will not be able to take it anymore, and will crash in the form of sickness, depression and anxiety. No one is a superhuman. We are all creations of nature, and nature is above all of us. We are products of nature and we can thrive when we live within its laws.

Unfortunately, sleep deprivation is not just limited to working professionals, but also to students. This is not to say that you should not make money, aim for high designations, or own fancy things. Have all of this, but with a parallel focus on health, and how you were meant to live, considering we are all products of nature. All of us have pulled all-nighters at some point in our lives, and that is not a problem. The problem arises when all-nighters start to become a common phenomenon and part of our lifestyle, leading to a chronic deprivation of sleep.

So, it is not about hustling your way to success. True success is when we can achieve all our goals and still maintain our physical and emotional health, a peaceful state of mind and happy relationships.

Even if we think we don't need sleep or skip sleep during the week thinking that we can cover the sleep debt over the weekend, our body doesn't care. What our body cares for is survival and it will do anything for that. And really, what is sickness? It is our body trying to slow us down. So there is no point in challenging nature and its perfectly designed circadian rhythm. Even the best treatment, medicines, doctors, nutritionists, spiritual healers or yoga experts will not work for a body that is sleep-deprived. The very process of healing, recovery, detoxification, repair, muscle growth and fat loss happens during sleep.

Having said that, yes, cases of insomnia and the inability to fall asleep no matter what, are real, but only a few cases like these are genuine. For everyone else, it's their lifestyle and habits that come in the way of the process of falling asleep naturally which has been explained in depth throughout this book.

The way I like to plan every day of my life is by knowing that I do not have 24 hours in a day. I have 24 minus 8 hours in a day, because those 8 hours are for my sleep and nothing can come between that. I then plan my work, workouts, family time, me time, entertainment, reading and study for the remaining 16 hours. Sleep is my lynchpin and I cannot function without it. And no, prioritising sleep doesn't mean giving up on all the fun and socialising. You can still socialise, but in a smart way. Half of the things we try to do in order to attain good health and great bodies may not even be required if we just focus on our sleep.

Because sleep is the most underrated tool for good health and longevity, and still it feels so elusive to many of us, I appreciate Khurshed Batliwala and Dinesh Ghodke for putting together this amazing book that addresses sleep and talks about necessary concepts like circadian rhythm, winding down and meditation so beautifully.

Sleep is one of my favourite subjects, and much of my work with patients revolves around this lifestyle pillar and trying to link sleep deprivation with the possible onset of a disease. The magic of sleep is powerful. It is one of the deepest meditations known, and no other drug or pill can ever replace it.

It has been an absolute pleasure to write this piece for your book. I wish you and this amazing book great success!

Luke Coutinho

SLEEP

Why Sleep

Thomas Lackey did wing-walking—stunts on the wing of an airplane while it is flying—at the age of 93! John Evans balanced a car—a Mini Cooper weighing around 160 kg—on his head for 33 seconds. Taking skydiving to a completely different level, Felix Baumgartner jumped from a helium balloon floating over the surface of the earth at 135,000 feet. He plummeted to the earth in free fall for over 4 minutes, reaching a top speed of around 1350 km/hr, becoming the first human to break the sound barrier without a vehicle. Yes, he wore something like a space suit and used a parachute towards the end. Michael Lotito ate—yes—ate an entire airplane, a Cessna 150. Jackie Bibby held 13 live rattlesnakes in his mouth.

The Guinness Book of World Records is home to these and many more astonishing, scary, daring and weird feats that we, as human beings, have performed.

But did you know that the *Guinness Book* doesn't allow records for staying awake? There were a few in earlier editions, but not anymore. The people who run the *Guinness Book* don't mind recording stuff about people holding live rattlesnakes in their mouth or eating an airplane, but they consider going without sleep to be 'too dangerous' and so, have banned the setting of any such records!

The Sleep Famine

Some of the biggest disasters in recent times—the Challenger Space Shuttle explosion, the Chernobyl meltdown, the Exxon Valdez oil spill—to name a few, have been attributed to lack of enough sleep. Staff who had been working 30-40 hour shifts just dozed off at critical moments.

We all know about drunken driving, and the appalling number of casualties it causes. There are tests, fines and laws for that in all countries. Did you know that around four times more accidents are caused because of something called 'Drowsy Driving'—falling asleep for a few seconds on the wheel? At 100 km/hr, 5 seconds could prove fatal. No country that I know of has any provision in their law for falling asleep while driving.

The US alone spends over $500 billion every year because of sleep deprivation and the related loss in productivity, creativity and efficiency.

Our bodies go through stages of sleep every night when we snooze. N1 and N2 are considered 'light sleep'. We go through the light sleep stage and enter the deeper stages, N3, N4 and REM. During N3/4 our bodies undergo major rejuvenation and repair work. This is when the brain is literally printing out our body for the next day. Not enough N3/4 and we age faster, our skin loses its lustre making us look older and uglier.

During REM, memories of the day are being transferred from short-term to long-term storage and the brain creates a sense of chronology. We dream. Somehow, our brain makes connections from all the stuff we know, leading to those elusive flashes of pure genius. Have you ever woken up with a brilliant idea? That's a gift of REM sleep. Not enough REM sleep makes us grow dumber and more forgetful.

The Cerebro Spinal Fluid (CSF), in which our brain floats, does a deep cleanse of the brain every night as we sleep. Through the course of the day, while doing all of its myriad activities, there is a particularly toxic chemical that our brain produces as waste, called Beta Amyloid. A buildup of Beta Amyloid is considered to be the leading cause of most brain degenerative diseases—Alzheimer's, Parkinson's, dementia … not enough sleep means you are giving an open invitation to these terrible conditions as you grow older. It's only when we sleep, that the spaces between brain cells increase by around 60% giving the CSF a chance to get in there and do a thorough mop up.

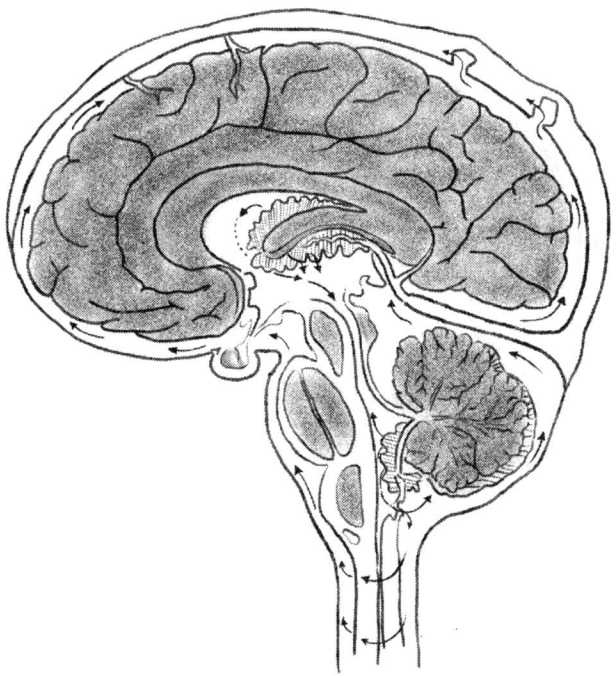

The arrows indicate the flow of the CSF in and around the brain

A study was done with a group of crack shot soldiers who typically had over 98% accuracy. When the number of hours they slept was reduced, their accuracy plummeted quite dramatically.

With 7+ hours of sleep, the soldiers had 98% accuracy.

6 hours of sleep got their accuracy down to 50%.

5 hours of sleep, and they just had 35% accuracy.

4 hours of sleep brought the accuracy of a highly skilled soldier down to just 15%.

Transpose this into your life and the things you do during the day. Think about how much more you could have accomplished if you had given yourself enough time to sleep.

Sleep Deprivation is Insidious

The biggest problem with sleep deprivation is that the person who is sleep deprived doesn't realise it.

For example, say you have had a full day at work and decide to hang out with friends in the evening. You lose track of time and suddenly realise that it's almost 1 a.m. You take your leave and drive home. At that point, your response to the road and traffic will be the same as a person who is over the legally drunk limit.

Yet, you will say you are fine and of course, you can drive home. A drunk person knows he is drunk. A sleep-deprived person hardly ever realises that he is sleep deprived. A coaching client of mine kept pushing himself to work harder and harder, managing and coping with very little sleep for months on end. He was driven to make his business succeed, and many times, he would work for 30+ hours straight. He said he would relax in the gym. He had a powerful physique and considered himself super fit.

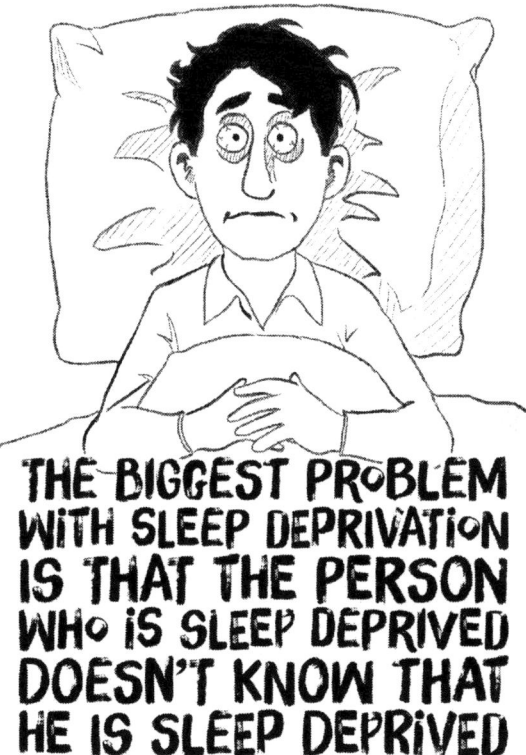

THE BIGGEST PROBLEM WITH SLEEP DEPRIVATION IS THAT THE PERSON WHO IS SLEEP DEPRIVED DOESN'T KNOW THAT HE IS SLEEP DEPRIVED

One day, he simply collapsed out of sheer exhaustion. Out of the blue, he had a panic attack that left him debilitated. He continued to suffer from anxiety and panic attacks for almost three years. Fortunately, he had hired good people and they ran his multimillion dollar business with minimal input from him as he slowly tried to recover from his affliction.

When he approached me for help, he told me that he wanted to be as he had been earlier. After hearing his story, I told him if he wanted to work with me, he would never be like he was earlier. That was what had caused all the problems in the first place. He had still not made the connection between what was going on with him and lack of sleep.

After working with him for a few months, and mainly fixing his sleep routine and his diet, he himself was astonished at how amazing he felt as he quickly recovered. He sleeps 8 hours every night now and has taken back control of his life as I write this.

Lack of sleep can lead to poor judgement. And poor judgement, in an instant can wipe out a career, reputation and wealth that may have taken decades to establish. Most critically, lack of sleep leads to poor judgement about how much sleep you should have. This can create a disastrous snowball effect that can create severely adverse effects on you, your family and your business or organisation you are working for.

Sleep-deprived people grow fat faster. Leptin is a hunger hormone that decreases appetite. Ghrelin is the other hunger hormone and it makes you feel hungry. When you don't sleep enough, ghrelin production spikes. You feel hungry all the time and crave mostly junk. To make it worse, when you are sleep-deprived, leptin production falls. This greatly magnifies your hunger pangs. Skimp on sleep and you are on your way to being well-rounded!

Research about sleep has shown that every single organ and system of the body is negatively impacted when you don't sleep enough. Lack of sleep translates to a host of unpleasant conditions like diabetes, heart disease, hypertension, mood disorders, learning disorders, stroke and compromised immunity. Deficiency of sleep will also rapidly kill your sex drive.

Less sleep lowers life expectancy. Worse, it severely compromises quality of life.

Conversely, if we sleep enough, we become healthier, more good looking, feel so much better about ourselves and develop a keener intellect.

I hope by now you are convinced that sleep is tremendously important. It's nature's gift to us to recharge, rejuvenate and recreate ourselves for the coming day. Please do yourself and others around you a favour—give yourself an 8-hour sleep opportunity each night.

Good Night!

The lark is silent in his nest,
The breeze is sighing in its flight,
Sleep, Love, and peaceful be thy rest.
Good night, my love, good night, good night.

Sweet dreams attend thee in thy sleep,
To soothe thy rest till morning's light,
And angels around thee vigil keep.
Good night, my love, good night, good night.

— Paul Laurence Dunbar

Three Questions

One of the biggest problems with sleep deprivation is not knowing that one is indeed sleep-deprived. Usually, people will have a breakdown or an accident before realising the havoc that lack of enough good quality sleep has wreaked on their systems.

Here are three questions you can ask yourself to figure out if you are getting enough high-quality sleep. If the answer to even one of these questions is in the negative, it means your time in bed is not optimised and you could be sleep-deprived—even though you may not feel it.

1. Do you wake up in the morning without an alarm?
If you wake up with an alarm, there are high chances that you are not getting all the sleep you require. We go through various stages of sleep—N1 and N2 are considered light sleep from where we transition to the deep sleep states of REM and N3/4. When we awaken, we move from N3/4 or REM into N2, then into N1, then to being fully awake.

An alarm could potentially yank us forcefully out of deep sleep to being fully awake in seconds. When an alarm rings, however pleasant sounding it is, your adrenaline levels suddenly spike as the brain registers what it can only understand as 'danger'. Your blood pressure abruptly shoots up and you awaken with assorted stress hormones flooding your system. If you usually hit the snooze button on the alarm and go back to sleep for another 5-10 minutes, then you are subjecting your body to another surge of stress when your alarm beeps yet again in a few minutes. This is a nasty way to wake up and most people who do so will feel grumpy and tired during the day.

In the worst-case scenario, habitually using the alarm clock to wake up could eventually lead to a heart attack or a stroke.

Get rid of that alarm clock. Sleep earlier if required, so that you wake up naturally and fully rested, feeling relaxed, easy and calm.

2. When you awaken each morning, do you feel refreshed, energised and rejuvenated?

A lot of people could wake up feeling disoriented and groggy. If this happens once in a while, that's alright. If it happens too often, then this is a clear indication that the quality (and quantity) of sleep they are getting is not good enough. There could be many reasons for this. In later chapters, we will explore ways of ensuring great quality sleep. Here is a quick checklist of some of the most common reasons why people could wake up tired even when they feel they have slept more than enough:

1. You didn't sleep for 8 to 10 hours. Sleeping less than 8 hours is detrimental to your body–mind complex. Give yourself an 8-hour sleep opportunity each night.
2. You take sleeping pills. These are a bad idea. There are no 'sleeping' pills actually available on the market. This medication merely sedates you. Sedation is not the same as sleep. When sedated, you get none of the benefits of natural sleep. Besides, these are habit-

forming and make you addicted to them and mess up other systems in your body. Wean yourself off them as soon as you can if you are taking them, always in consultation with whoever recommended them to you in the first place. A good ayurvedic or homeopathic doctor can help. I have seen Craniosacral Therapy combined with Bach Flower Therapy yield amazing results.

3. Some types of medication that you are taking could interfere with sleep.
4. You ate your last meal just before going to bed. Eat an early dinner. Give yourself at least 3 hours between your dinner and sleep.
5. You have light in the bedroom. Even tiny lights can disrupt sleep. Black out your bedroom.
6. Bright lights in the bathroom could be to blame for disturbed sleep. It's okay to go to the loo in the middle of the night if you need to. What's not okay are the bright lights in the bathroom which can signal the brain to start the wake cycle, making it difficult to go back to bed.
7. You had coffee or tea towards late evening, or you are having too many cups of coffee and/or tea in a day. The caffeine in these beverages mess up your sleep rhythm.
8. You had alcohol. Alcohol will interfere with normal sleep cycles and play havoc with your brain. You may get knocked out by having too much alcohol, but that is not to be confused with sleep.
9. You exercised vigorously after 8 p.m. Vigorous exercise may release hormones like adrenaline into your blood stream. This increases your heart rate, makes the brain active, and raises the core body temperature, all of

which as a Harvard study blithely puts it, may keep you up at night 'hooting with the owls'!
10. You slept too much during the day. Do not take a power nap of more than 30 minutes in the afternoon.
11. You are anxious or excited about something in your life. Practise yoga and meditation to relax the body and soothe the mind. You will sleep much better.
12. You are sleeping in a new place. You may have noticed that when you go on a holiday, the first night or two you may not get good sleep. This is natural. It's an evolutionary response from deep within the brain. The brain needs to be convinced that there is no danger in the environment before allowing the body to switch off completely. Meditation, chanting and keeping a few familiar things in the room would help.
13. Your room could be too hot or too cold.
14. There is too much noise in the surroundings, or your bedroom could be too quiet.
15. The air quality of your bedroom is not very good.
16. The clothes you are wearing to sleep are uncomfortable or tight.
17. Your bed and pillows are uncomfortable.
18. Of course, if you are just plain unwell—you have a blocked nose or you injured your foot and that's hurting a lot, sleep could be compromised—though hopefully that's just a temporary thing.

3. Does this feeling of being refreshed last until 12 noon?
There is a natural sleep pressure build up in our systems towards afternoon. By 2 p.m. most people will feel sleepy. This is natural and is a great time to take a nap of around 30 minutes. A Yoga-Nidra meditation would be perfect. A quick nap will refresh you and keep you energised for the evening ahead.

However, if you are feeling tired and sleepy before 12 in the afternoon, it again means that your sleep is compromised and you need to actively do something about it. We will explore a lot of points on the list above throughout this book. Even if your answer to all the three questions is a yes, go over the list and see if any of them are relevant to you.

Small changes can create big gains and better sleep will ultimately translate into a better you.

What small change regarding your sleeping habits are you going to make tonight?

Good Night!

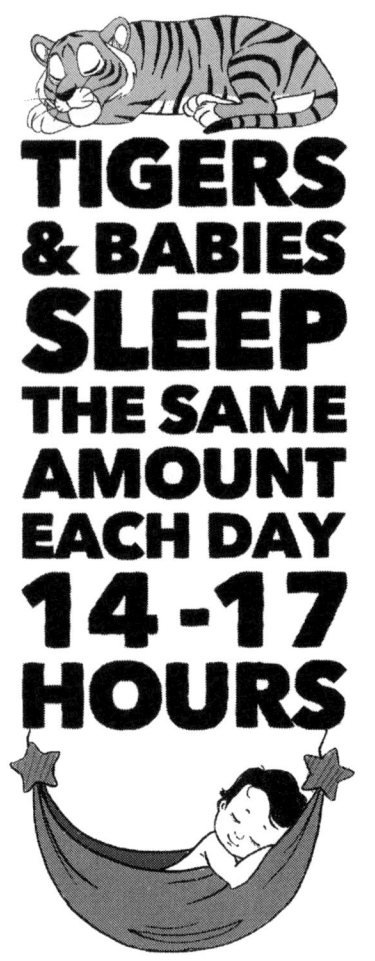

Falling Asleep

Do you notice how you habitually feel hungry at certain times of the day? Or feel tired at other times? Or how during a particular time period in the day you are most productive? And then there are times when you just want to chill and relax.

My productive period is in the morning from around 9 a.m. to 1 p.m. and then again in the evening from 7 p.m. to 9 p.m. I love to catch a quick nap around 2 p.m. and relax after 9 p.m. I am hungriest at around 10 a.m. I am a different person at different times of the day—and so are you.

You change physiologically as well through the day. There are times when your body temperature is high and other times when it is low (varies by around 1.5 degrees through a 24-hour time period). Your blood pressure, heart rate, digestion rate and countless other parameters will fluctuate throughout the day. Notice how your potty time is approximately the same time each day. Though you may go to urinate quite a few times during the day, you have almost no urge to pee during the 8 hours you sleep at night.

Ever wondered how our bodies keep time? How does the body know it's time for lunch, or time to meditate or sleep or work or play? How does it know when to make you feel sleepy and when to allow you to focus and concentrate?

You may look at a watch and say it's 6.45 in the evening. This doesn't mean that your body knows that the time is 6.45 in the evening. The body has its own highly sophisticated mechanism to tell time.

The Circadian Rhythm

Every single cell in your body has a clock. These miniscule clocks operate on a more or less 24-hour rhythm. To coordinate between all those millions and millions of molecular clocks, there is a master clock—a tiny group of cells deep inside your brain called the Suprachiasmatic Nucleus (SCN). The SCN gets cues from daylight and the darkness of the night to figure out what time of the day or night it is. Additionally, the SCN decides what time it is depending on when you eat your meals. This enables all those millions of clocks all over the body to be synchronised with each other, and maintain healthy circadian rhythms. 'Circadian' means recurring naturally over a 24-hour cycle.

Through evolution, for millions of years, light and food were extremely reliable cues … until our modern society happened almost in a flash. Suddenly, artificial light vandalised the darkness of the night, and all types of food came to be available at all times. Now, the SCN has to deal with conflicting cues from the environment.

The sun has set; the SCN has distinctly registered this, yet there is bright white and blue light, not the warm oranges and yellows of fire that it would have expected to perceive to signify that night has begun Irregular meal times compound this confusion. All this baffles the SCN and throws it out of whack, resulting in what is called 'circadian disruption'. Essentially, your body no longer knows what time it really is, and cannot figure out whether it's time to sleep, stay awake, do work, play, relax, digest food, excrete, raise or lower blood pressure and heartbeat ... you get the idea.

This may sound amusing—a confused body clock—but it can become quite a health challenge. Take shift workers for example. For their bodies, the light and dark cues become utterly bewildering, considerably increasing their risks of developing all sorts of cancers. The WHO (World Health Organisation) actually lists working in shifts as a carcinogen.

Jet lag is another big disruption of the circadian rhythm. Anyone who has done long-distance air travel has experienced some of the symptoms of jet lag—exhaustion, difficulty staying awake and being alert during the day, inability to fall asleep at night, loss of memory, gastrointestinal issues, heaviness in the head, a feeling of being unwell, etc.

Our bodies didn't evolve to fly at high speeds around the world. For each hour your body travels through a time zone, it requires a full day to recalibrate itself. Fly from Mumbai to London, and you move through 5 to 6 time zones. Your body will need almost a week to completely resynchronise all the internal clocks and start feeling normal again.

Social Jet Lag

Finally, it's Friday.

After a long hard week of work, all you want to do in the evening is be at home and chill and unwind with a few good friends. You watch a movie, gossip, have dinner, gossip some more, play a board game or two, all the time munching on some snack or the other ... and it is 2 a.m. before everyone calls it a night and you finally get into bed to catch some sleep. You then tend to sleep in late on Saturday, eat a late breakfast, an even later lunch and an almost midnight dinner. Possibly repeat the same sequence on Saturday night and

Sunday, with minor variations ... sounds like a fabulous weekend, doesn't it?

The abnormal light and dark cues—sleeping late means too much light at night, waking up late means your body registers sunrise much later than it usually does. Factor in the snacking and your SCN and other body clocks get as muddled as if you have been on a long-distance flight.

The weekend is over and on Monday, you feel exhausted, a little disoriented, don't feel like getting out of bed, forget stuff, can't focus too well—all symptoms of jet lag. Monday morning blues is just jet lag without even stepping onto an airplane.

A vast majority of people around the world repeat this pattern week after week, month after month, habitually disrupting their circadian rhythms which are physiologically linked to every single organ and system of the body. They end up chronically jet lagged without ever leaving home.

This dramatically increases the risk of all sorts of unpleasant health conditions—from hypertension, diabetes and depression to cancers and dementia.

The easiest way to avoid all this nastiness is:
1. Get plenty of morning sunlight. The SCN gets its light cues from your eyes, so remember not to wear sunglasses when you take a morning walk. 15 minutes to half an hour of direct sunlight is fantastic.
2. Exposure to sunlight a few times during the day is highly recommended.
3. No bright lights in the evening, from around 3 hours before bedtime. Switch off lights that are not being used and dim others. Watching the sunset, as the whites and blues of daylight fade into yellows, oranges and pinks of dusk and then

to the darkness is one of the best things you can do for your SCN.
4. Sleep and wake up at around the same time every day—even on weekends.

Why am I making such a big deal about the SCN and light in a book about sleep and success?

Well, depending on cues from the environment, the SCN regulates the sleep–wake circadian cycle. Towards evening, as it registers the approach of night, the SCN triggers the release of melatonin, which in turn sets into motion all the bodily mechanisms for orchestrating sleep.

Close your eyes and you will realise that you can still 'feel' light. This is how the SCN recognises that the night is over and initiates the secretion of cortisol which rouses you from drowsiness, sets systems in motion to make you alert and gets your body ready for the day ahead. For the people who feel they just have to have their morning cuppa—know that cortisol (and adrenaline) are ten times stronger than anything caffeine can do to make you feel awake each morning.

This melatonin–cortisol dance is coordinated by the SCN—see the graph above on how melatonin and cortisol levels fluctuate through the day and night.

If your SCN cannot tell the time, you will not be able to sleep easily, deeply or enough, nor will you feel refreshed and alert through the day. This will dramatically impact quality of life as we have seen earlier. However, keeping your SCN happy is just one part of the story of falling asleep and waking up.

Adenosine

During digestion, the glucose in your food breaks down a couple of times, forming many fancy-sounding chemicals, names that we will not get into. Eventually, it transforms into adenosine. Through the day, the adenosine levels rise steadily in the bloodstream. Adenosine interacts with specific neural receptors and causes drowsiness by inhibiting neural activity.

The higher the adenosine level in the blood, the drowsier you will feel. In this way, adenosine produces an impetus within you to want to sleep. This impetus gets stronger and stronger as you stay awake longer and longer.

This impetus is called 'Sleep Drive' or 'Sleep Pressure' and is completely independent of the machinations of the SCN.

When you sleep, the adenosine molecules are flushed away from the neural receptors they were occupying. As this happens, the inhibition on neural activity is slowly released, and as sleep pressure is lifted, you wake up. This 'Sleep War' continues in your body—one part of you compelling you to fall asleep, the other bent on keeping you awake.

It's worth noting that the sleep drive makes you sleepy—not tired. You may feel tired because of mental and/or physical exhaustion, but that may not necessarily make you feel sleepy.

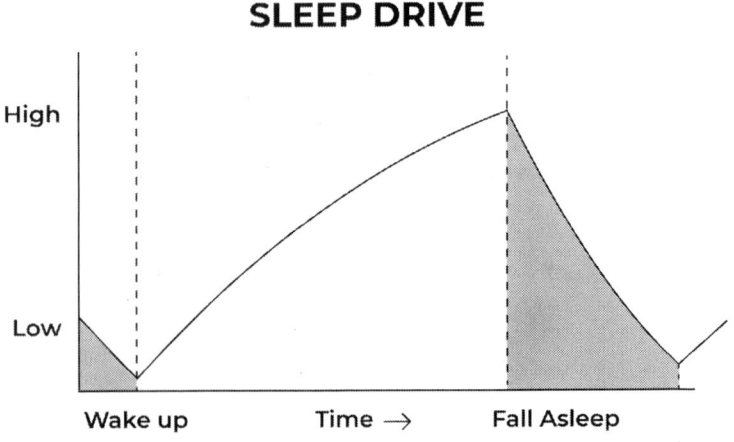

The Effects of Coffee

Coffee is a stimulant addictive drug—check out the effects of coffee on spiders weaving their webs compared to some other drugs in the illustration below. This was part of some obscure research conducted by NASA in the 1980s. There is no need for any comment once you see the image. For the moment, let's keep this shady side of coffee aside and look at what having just one cup of coffee does to our systems.

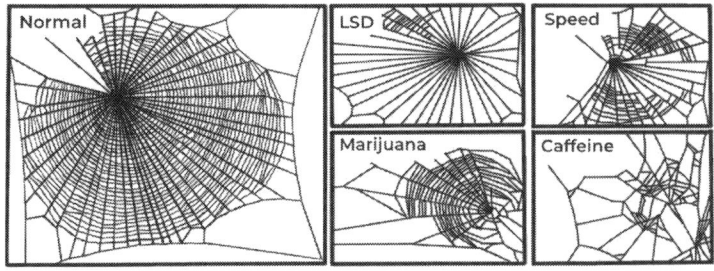

Effects of Various Drugs on Spider Web Building

The caffeine molecule is similar to the adenosine molecule. When you drink coffee (or anything else that has caffeine in it), you flood your system with caffeine molecules which promptly go and occupy the neural receptors reserved for adenosine. This means that even though there is an adenosine build-up in the blood, the neural receptors don't register it. Your body is crying, 'I want sleep!' Yet the coffee stifles its screams, and so you experience the illusion of feeling awake and alert.

It takes your body approximately 8 hours to nullify the effect of one cup of coffee. Avoid drinking coffee after 2 in the afternoon—only then will there be enough sleep pressure build up by 10 or 11 p.m. to warrant going to bed.

And if you do drink tea or coffee, don't have it first thing in the morning, as most people do. At this time, anyway there is no adenosine around to keep you from feeling drowsy. Have your coffee between 10 and 11 a.m.—this will help you to overcome the afternoon slump in alertness and still not interfere with your nightly sleep.

The effect of caffeine to delay and suppress sleep is much stronger than that of bright light at night. Also, caffeine is a diuretic and will make you want to pee. So when you do fall asleep, the pressure to pee will wake you up and disturb your sleep. Remember this and those spiders weaving their webs and never have more than two cups of coffee in a day, and definitely no coffee towards the evening or night.

Sleep

Sleeping (and waking) is a function of the dance between the two systems—sleep drive and the circadian rhythm. The sleep drive makes you feel progressively sleepy through the day. The SCN, as part of the circadian rhythm, will perceive the onset of night through visual cues and release melatonin to begin the preparation for the body to fall asleep.

When both these systems peak, a fantastic doorway into sleep is created—see the image below. It's best to start your winding down ritual during this time. You will effortlessly slip into deep restful sleep.

In much the same way, a beautiful doorway to wake up is created in the morning as the circadian rhythm signals squirts of cortisol to rouse you from slumber, and the pressure of the sleep drive has been almost nullified. Waking up during this time, and not spending the usual 15 minutes to an hour lolling around in bed will make you feel awake, alert and refreshed for the greater part of the day. It is best if you can get out of bed within 5 minutes of waking up. Trust me, the rest of the day will feel brighter and you will be able to get so much more done.

The 'what a beautiful morning' feeling will last till approximately 12 in the afternoon, by which time the adenosine accumulation will make you feel drowsy again.

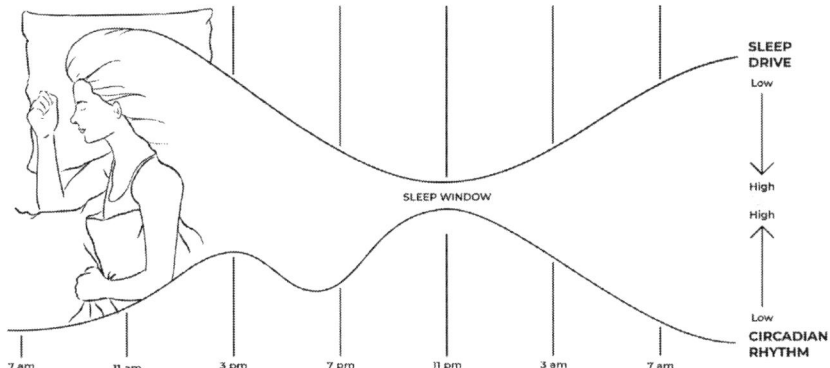

A short nap of around 20-30 minutes is enough to flush out the adenosine, and keep you awake and alert till late evening. Not catching a quick power nap in the afternoon might build sleep pressure and keep you from being alert and awake through the rest of the day.

If you want to maximise the efficiency of this power nap, time it between 2 and 3 p.m. After lunch, your blood sugar and energy levels will take a dip and taking a quick 20-minute nap at this time is highly recommended.

Benefits of an afternoon nap include:
1. Enhanced learning ability, especially right after the nap
2. Improved performance and productivity
3. Lower blood pressure and decreased risk of cardiovascular disease (by as much as 20%)
4. Better mood as you are less irritable

Be careful with the napping, though. If you nap for more than 30 minutes,

1. You may wake up feeling drowsy, disoriented, sluggish and perhaps even more tired than you felt before the nap—definitely not as alert and refreshed as you might hope to be.
2. It might become difficult for you to fall asleep easily at night.

Studies indicate that naps longer than an hour in the afternoon significantly increase the risk of heart disease and dying. The only exception to this is if you are sleep-deprived and have the time to be able to complete a full sleep cycle of approximately 90 minutes as you nap in the afternoon.

A robust circadian rhythm, a healthy sleep drive and a 20-minute nap between 2 and 3 p.m. will ensure the right amount of deep restful sleep every night and a feeling of freshness and alertness throughout the day.

Stages of Sleep

We often say, 'I slept really well', or 'I had really good sleep'. Is there good sleep and bad sleep? Deep sleep and light sleep?

Turns out there is.

I was playing with my dog Bobby. We were running around the garden, wrestling with each other, playing tag, throwing and fetching stuff. Bobby is a small dog and all that exercise must have tired him out. When we got home, he jumped on to our sofa—his favourite place to nap—and went to sleep.

I took a bath and freshened up and saw something quite strange. Though Bobby was fast asleep, his eyeballs under his closed eyelids were moving furiously. He seemed to be smiling. I called out his name a few times, but all I got was a tiny wag from his tail. I called Mom and showed her what was happening. She smiled and said, 'He is dreaming.'

She was absolutely spot on.

That movement of eyeballs when we are fast asleep happens to everyone, and to many animals as well. It was first noticed by Eugene Aserinsky, a graduate student at the University of Chicago in 1952. He was studying patterns of eye movements in human infants. He noticed periods of energetic movement, intertwined with long periods when the eyes would be calm and at rest. Further, he saw that the animated eye movement was accompanied by a spike in brain wave activity.

Professor Nathaniel Kleitman, his mentor, wanted to see if this phenomenon was replicable and chose his own daughter Ester to check if Aserinsky's findings were indeed accurate.

They were.

And REM sleep was discovered. REM stands for 'Rapid Eye Movement'. This is the time we all dream.

With classic scientific creativity, the duo named the calm periods of sleep 'NREM'—Non-REM sleep.

NREM was further classified into four stages:

- N1: When you are just dozing off, but you are hazily aware of what's going on around you. If you asked someone if they came into the room while you were obviously asleep and they expressed surprise saying, 'How did you know? You were fast asleep', you were probably in N1 or the beginning of N2.
- N2: You are asleep. From here, you can transition into the deeper sleep of N3 and N4 or go into REM.
- N3 and N4: These are the stages of really deep restful rejuvenating sleep.

All the NREM sleep stages had specific brainwave patterns that allowed sleep researchers to identify which stage someone was in. They found that a healthy person would experience cycles of sleep each night. They would go from

N1 to N2. From N2, they would either go into N3/4 or REM. From N3/4 or REM, they could sequence back into N2 or N1 to a few seconds of actually waking up. And this cycle would repeat itself. For most adults, each sleep cycle is 90 minutes, give or take a few. Healthy adults need to have at least 5 sleep cycles from the time they hit the bed to the time they wake up.

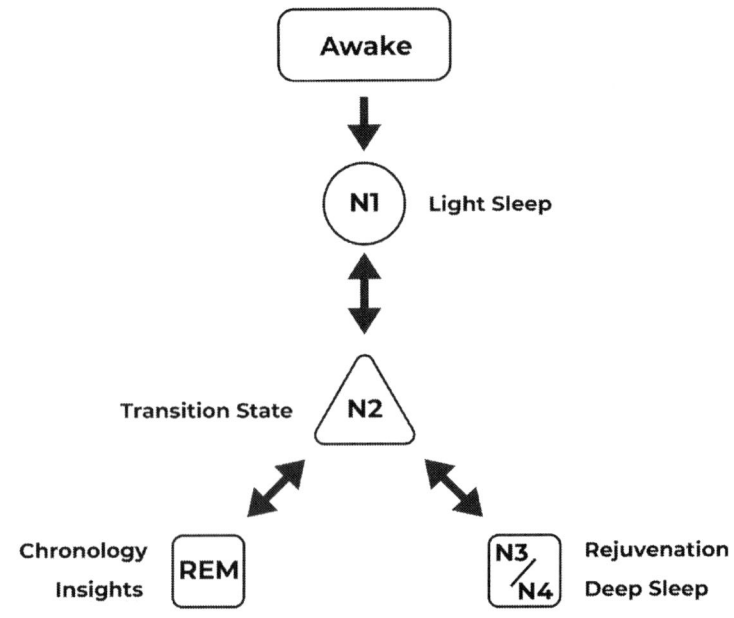

If you plot the different stages of sleep a person experiences throughout the night, then you would get a graph that looks something like this:

This graph is called a Hypnogram.

Look at the hypnogram closely, and you will see that towards the beginning of the night, you sleep more in N3/4 with hardly any REM. As the night gives way to the day, there is quite a lot of REM and very little N3/4.

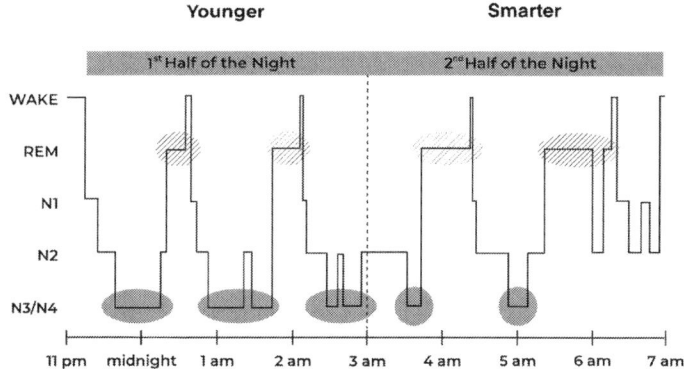

During REM sleep, your brain is quite active. The REM sleep brainwaves are quite similar to the waves produced by the brain when you are awake. N3 and N4 sleep waves are slow, sweeping all over the brain.

Making Movies

My friend Gowrishankar, who makes short films, once told me an astounding fact about making movies. He stated that they shot almost 200 times more footage than what actually makes it into the final cut of a feature film.

Once the shooting is done, the movie goes into the editing room, where the real magic happens. They go over all the material and make big cuts of stuff that then does not make it to the film. At the same time, they also tweak and adjust sequences that are likely to be in the film. They do this a few times until they have whittled down everything to what will almost certainly be in the final film.

Then it's all about polishing the film, often even making microsecond corrections that brings the film together to hopefully become the next blockbuster hit.

Our brain does much the same thing with our memories while we sleep.

In the early parts of the night, during N3/4 stages, it is shaving down the impressions of the near past and deciding what parts of our memory are going to be deleted and what parts preserved for long-term storage from the tenuous short-term centres they are stored in. The N3/4 stages act as the first big cuts in the editing process, wherein the brain deletes whole swathes of what it considers fairly useless pieces of information (what you had for lunch last Thursday, or what was the last OTP you used, for example). The short bursts of REM sleep at that time are for making the finer adjustments to the memories the brain has decided to keep.

Towards morning, during REM sleep, the brain is busy integrating the memories it decided to preserve of the near past with those of your more distant past. This is what gives you a sense of chronology and you know which events happened earlier or later than the others. This is the time you dream—perhaps the brain is playing out its latest movie for your entertainment.

While these memory sortings are going on, the brain has to integrate newer information without losing the older information. Inside the brain, this translates into huge masses of neurons slithering and sliding into place, creating millions of new connections, while maintaining older connections. Many a time, serendipity strikes—and you wake up with a brilliant idea or a really cool solution to a sticky problem you might be dealing with.

The neural activity during REM sleep will create coherence from all the information you have been exposed to during the day. You will understand more of what you learned when you awaken after a full night's rest.

REM sleep makes you smarter.

N3/4 sleep is restful and rejuvenating for the body. Your body enters an 'under construction' mode as it repairs and replenishes the organs, muscles and systems. There is a humungous amount of complicated chemistry we routinely do in our sleep. It is sufficient to understand that N3/4 sleep is the time when your brain is literally 'printing out' your body for the next day. If you get enough N3/4 sleep, you wake up feeling refreshed and invigorated, excited for the day ahead. Your skin becomes silky smooth, your face glows, you look and feel younger. Your immune system is regenerated. You become healthier. Every single system of the body is positively impacted with enough N3/4 sleep.

Conversely, not enough N3/4 sleep will mean that your brain does a shoddy job of printing out your body for the next day. Every single system of your body is adversely, and sometimes irreversibly, affected. You wake up feeling tired and irritable. You feel much older than you are and age faster. You are more prone to falling sick. Inevitably, your youthful looks suffer.

How much Sleep?

N3/4 sleep will make you younger, healthier and sexier. REM Sleep makes you smarter and provides you with a sense of chronology. Together, N3/4 sleep and REM sleep makes your memory stronger and provide you with flashes of insights and ideas.

Sleep is nature's superpower which, when invoked, will make you younger, healthier, smarter and sexier. Don't sleep enough and you will grow older, uglier and dumber.

The question then is, how much sleep is enough sleep?

As stated previously, adults need at least 5 sleep cycles, approximately 8 hours of sleep each night. Here is a chart for optimal sleep requirements for various age groups:

Let's say you normally sleep at 11 p.m. and wake up at 7 a.m., and clock in your full sleep requirement. If, for example, you sleep an hour later—you might think you just missed

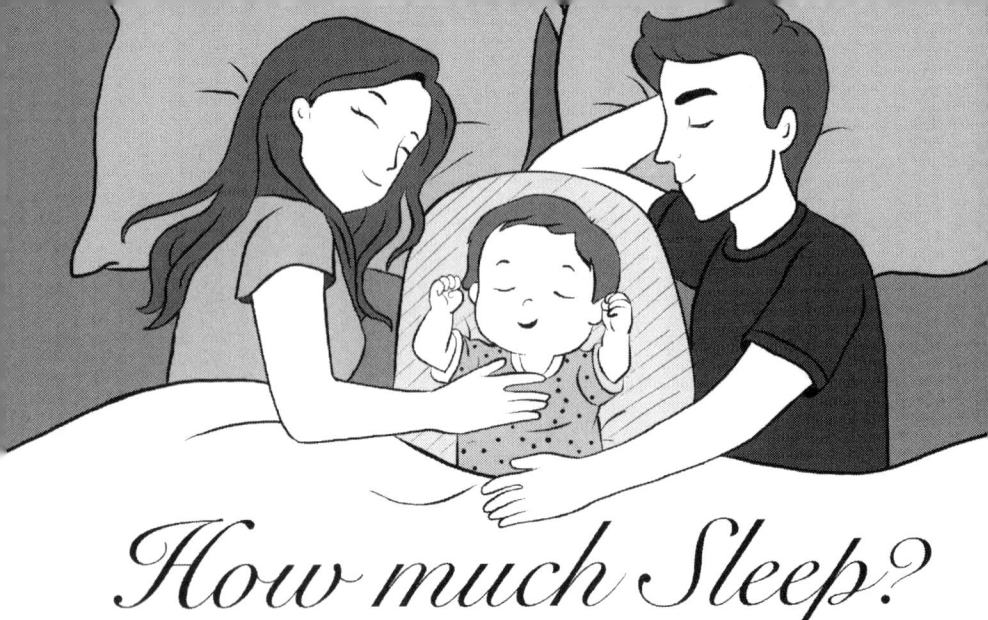

How much Sleep?

New Borns (0-3 months) **14-17 hours**

Infants (4-11 months) **12-15 hours**

Toddlers (1-2 years) **11-14 hours**

Pre-schoolers (3-5 years) **10-13 hours**

Children (6-13 years) **9-11 hours**

Teens (14-17 years) **8-10 hours**

Adults (18-65 years) **7-9 hours**

Older Adults (65+ years) **7-8 hours**

about 12.5% of your daily sleep requirement. However, if you look at the hypnogram, you will see you missed out on around 25% of your NREM sleep—for that night, you have aged faster than you should have.

Similarly, if you wake up an hour earlier, you will end up compromising more than 25% of your REM sleep for that night. You will feel disoriented and sluggish that day.

It is possible to pay off this sleep debt, but it needs to be done over a period of a few days, and you only have a short window of opportunity to do it. Life happens and you might miss an hour or two of sleep. Then, over the next week or so, sleep for about 20 minutes more than usual and that sleep debt will be paid off. Sleeping for a few hours extra over the weekend to make up for lost sleep will not work. In fact, as we saw earlier, this will cause social jet lag. You cannot postpone paying off this sleep debt a few months into the future either. It needs to be done right away—within approximately 10 days.

There is a fantastic hack to help and it is called meditation. We will explore the relationship between sleep and meditation in the next chapter.

Sleep well and enough and everything will be better.

Good Night!

Sleep

Many think their sleep is an epic time waste,
Life would be better off, if sleep was erased.

Yet truth of its need, science is now finding,
How critical is the body's nightly unwinding.

Sloppy sleep will add inches to your waist,
Dull your glow, and draw you dumb-faced.

Lack of good rest tires body, slows the brain
Makes the next day feel mediocre and mundane.

Overall, bad sleep in winter, rain or summer,
Can make you feel uglier, older and dumber.

Get this book, read it, enjoy it, gift it,
Also to the string of sleep hacks commit …

You'll learn about sleep's power and its mystery,
Your affair with your bed—can re-right history.

Smile and sleep your way to success true,
Sculpt a beautiful, youthful 'n smarter you!

— **Dinesh Ghodke**

Sleep and Meditation

Almost thirty years ago, I got bulldozed into doing an Art of Living course. It is something that I am forever grateful for.

In the course, I learned to meditate. It is the greatest of all adventures. It is the adventure inside of you.

You have probably gone on some of those wild escapades around the world. You might have experienced the rush of being on the world's fastest or twistiest rollercoaster, or felt the thrill of white water rafting on the Ganga, or done some serene, yet exciting, paragliding or parasailing. Maybe you have even been in a rocket and on the International Space Station or out in space … But let me tell you, the real adventure begins when you close your eyes and start meditating.

The feeling cannot be put in words, so I will not even try. Enough to say that if you have not learned to meditate, you are missing out on something beyond anything you can imagine or experience.

There are thousands of meditation techniques—some brilliant, others not a patch on the real thing. I would recommend that you learn and then stick to one technique. You cannot cross a river in two boats. Best to choose one boat and stick with it for the entire journey.

I have learned only the Art of Living techniques as taught by Gurudev Sri Sri Ravi Shankar and practised them for almost three decades. I can completely vouch for those. Not having studied any other form of meditation, and never having felt the need to, I cannot authentically comment on any other technique.

Don't try to learn meditation from a book—you can't. And meditation apps don't teach you how to meditate either, though they do manage to bring about some sort of relaxation within you. But relaxation is just the first thing that you will experience when you begin your meditation.

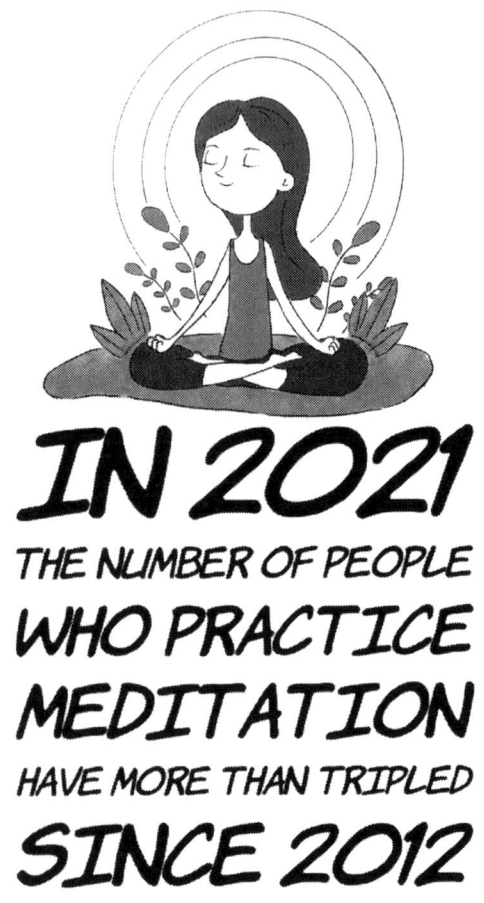

IN 2021 THE NUMBER OF PEOPLE WHO PRACTICE MEDITATION HAVE MORE THAN TRIPLED SINCE 2012

A well-researched, bona fide set of techniques like those from the Art of Living are highly recommended—you can find more details on **www.artofliving.org** and if you wish to learn these techniques with Dinesh, me and our team, you can check out our course schedules and enroll for them from **www.inergyworld.com**.

There has been tremendous amount of research around meditation and almost every single study shows how regular meditation will bring a whole range of incredible benefits. The brain of a meditator is physically different from the brain of a person who doesn't meditate. The ability to handle and process stress is greatly enhanced and the ability to enjoy life is magnified.

A meditator is fundamentally a more resilient, nicer person than a person who doesn't meditate. Meditation gives you a chance to become the best version of yourself.

Close Your Eyes …

If you are reading this, you are probably awake.

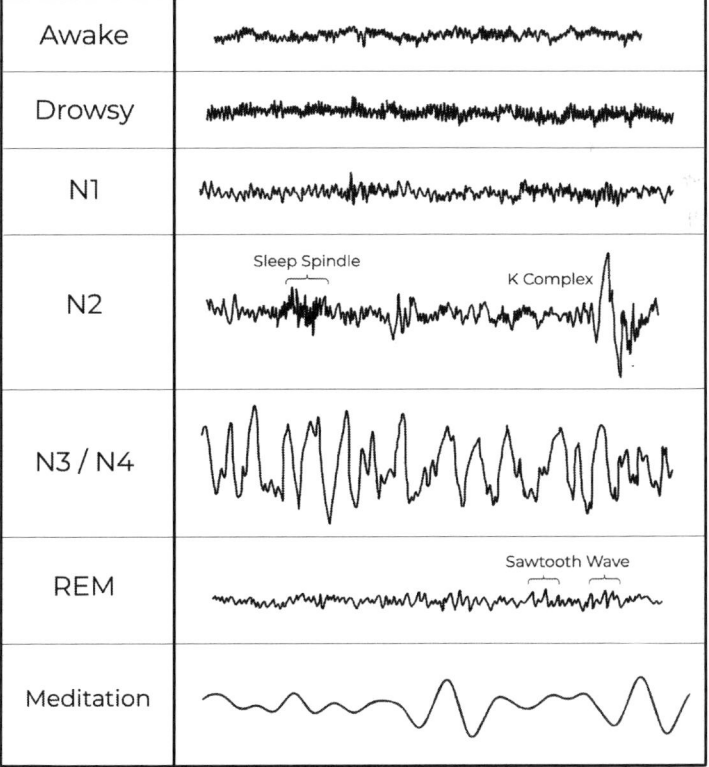

By reading this book, I hope you will be able to sleep better and have lovely dreams. And not stop there, but manifest your dreams into reality. And I hope by now, you feel inspired to learn and practise meditation as well.

There is a vast difference between sleep and mediation—though both begin with us closing our eyes. The brain waves of a person who is awake, sleeping, dreaming or meditating are remarkably different.

The Rishis broadly classified consciousness into four states:

Awake

Sleep

Dream

Meditative

The EEG brain waves seem to agree with their classification—the 4 states show up as pretty distinct patterns of electrical activity in the brain.

The electrical activity is different, because what the body and brain are accomplishing at each time are different.

As we saw earlier, what happens during states N1 to N4—rest and rejuvenation—is different from what happens during REM (or dream) state—chronology and insights. This means that what gets done when you are sleeping is quite different from what gets done when you are dreaming, even though most of the time we clump sleeping and dreaming together.

And of course, what you can accomplish when you are awake is different from what happens when you are asleep or dreaming.

Being in the meditative state is as natural as being awake, asleep or dreaming. Yet what happens during meditation is utterly different from the other three states. They are all different and serve different purposes.

In some ancient texts, it is mentioned that if you meditate for an hour, the freshness you feel will be like you have slept for 10 hours. Many people have made the mistake of misinterpreting this—assuming that if they meditate, they don't need to sleep as much as a person who doesn't meditate.

They then cut down their sleeping time to as little as four or five hours each night and end up damaging their bodies and minds. They set an alarm to wake up at 4 a.m. so that they can meditate. They are rudely yanked awake by their alarms and sit to meditate, only to fall asleep. The violent waking up each morning with an alarm can have long-term health risks—higher blood pressure, increased rate of cardiac problems, anxiety and even stroke. Couple this with chronically disturbed sleep every morning and a few years down the line, they develop all sorts of unpleasantness in their bodies and minds and wonder why all that is happening to them even though they meditate.

Thinking that meditation is a substitute for sleep is as foolish as thinking staying awake is an alternative to sleep. No one state of consciousness can ever be a substitute for another.

Having said all this, there are a few bonuses that people who meditate every day enjoy.

In a previous chapter, we had talked about sleep debt and how you need to pay it off within a few days. The window of how long you have to pay off sleep debt increases for a meditator.

People who regularly meditate will have deeper sleep—meaning they will not spend as much time in N1 and N2 as a normal person does and slip much faster into N3/4 or REM. In effect, they get a better deal with the same amount of sleep. And in case you are thinking, 'Aha! That means I don't need to sleep as much!', think again. Like everyone else, a meditator too needs his five sleep cycles. Just that those cycles do him much more good in terms of all the benefits of sleep than for someone who doesn't meditate—but the benefits are not enough for them to be able to afford to skip an entire cycle.

Regular meditators have pleasant dreams. Their meditation will normally delete all the unpleasant stuff from the mind.

Regular meditators can quickly adapt to a new space for sleeping. Have you noticed when you go someplace new for a vacation or a business trip, you don't get good sleep for the first day or two? It's an evolutionary response from the brain—it detects unfamiliar surroundings and so will not let you fall deeply asleep, just in case there is danger. A person who meditates typically will not have this problem, because meditation makes their nervous system far more robust, and the brain doesn't get easily alarmed.

Jet lag doesn't affect a meditator as much and your body clock is quick to recalibrate itself. After a long-distance flight, as a meditator, you will find it much easier to sleep and be fully rested much sooner than anyone would believe possible—especially if you meditated on the flight.

Sleep is primarily a function of various hormones in our body. Meditation optimally systemises the rise and fall of these hormones resulting in enriched sleep quality.

In fact, most of the emotional responses that stop sleep from happening—worry, fear, anxiety, depression, sadness, loneliness, anger, etc.—settle down when one meditates, and so sleep becomes effortless.

Good quality of sleep will deepen your meditation. Deep meditation will enhance your sleep. Both of these together will create heaven for you when you are awake.

Sleep. Meditate. Be happy. Make others around you happy.

Good Night!

The Bedroom

We humans are creatures of habit and habitat.
We do certain things in certain places. We go to a temple (or a fire temple, church, gurudwara, etc.) to worship. We go to a restaurant to dine or party. To a mall to shop. To a park or a garden to take a walk. To a gym to exercise. Most people cannot even think of doing anything else at each of these places.

In our homes too, certain rooms are for particular activities—the kitchen to cook, the hall to meet people and socialise, the study to well … study, and so on. Would you think of cooking in the bathroom? Or studying in the kitchen? Most definitely not. Yet, the bedroom is often invaded for a host of other activities. People watch TV, do their work, meet their friends … in their bedrooms. It would be best to reserve the bedroom for sleep, sex and sadhana (meditation).

Transform your bedroom into a sleep haven. A place that beckons you alluringly at the end of a day where you surrender everything and drift off into the enchanted wonderland of sleep.

Your very own personal, private space.

The Bedroom Makeover

In a nutshell, your bedroom should be cozy, cool, comfortable and pitch dark at night. You need to remove anything that is

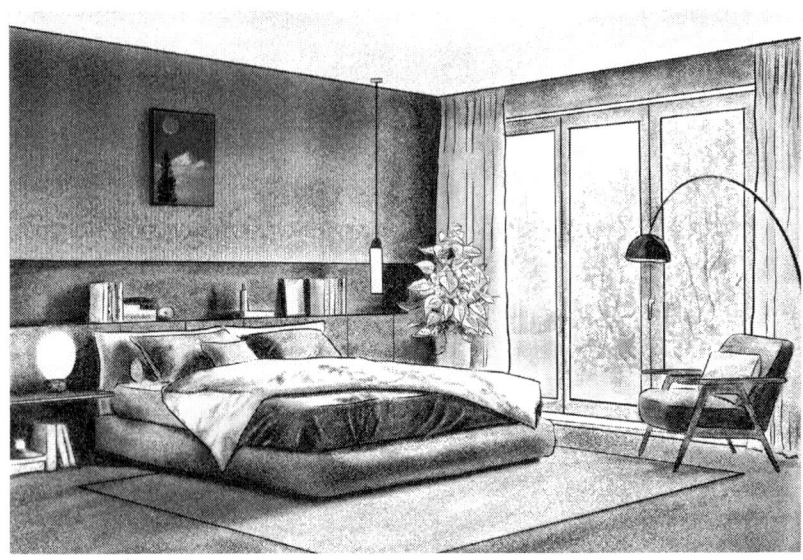

not relevant for sleep, while bringing in all the things that will encourage a great night's rest.

I remember my hostel room in IIT. For quite some time, it was a mess. Everything higgledy-piggledy everywhere. Washed clothes, unwashed clothes, textbooks, music CDs, magazines, chocolate wrappers—all over the place. When I wanted to study, I would just make some space in the mess and get down to it. And often I collapsed into whatever space was available to sleep.

Once I did the Art of Living series of programmes and learned to meditate, I was compelled to clean up my space. I loved meditation and it just didn't feel right to meditate in that cluttered and dirty space. So, one weekend, I emptied my room and scrubbed it from top to bottom with soap and water. My friends wondered if my mom was coming to visit.

It was a very small room. I had a bed, a study table, a minuscule bookshelf and a tiny cupboard. When I looked at the pile of random artifacts outside my room, I was quite taken aback at how much junk I had managed to accumulate. Methodically, I sorted out everything—what was precious, what I wanted to keep, what was not required, what I would give away and what I would simply junk. This was a long time before Marie Kondo—only I didn't write a book about it. Then I decided where everything went in the room. My mom used to always say, 'Everything in its place and a place for everything.' For the first time in my life, I appreciated the wisdom of what I had been hearing her say for twenty-odd years.

I took my time arranging things exactly the way I wanted them to be. When I finished, my room was transformed. Clean curtains, no cobwebs, new bedsheets, candles, Gurudev's photo with a fresh hibiscus flower in a little glass bowl near it and my study table elegantly organised. Now my bookshelf actually had books on it, not dirty underwear, and my cupboard wasn't a public hazard anymore. From then on, I kept my space clean and tidy, and I found that I could meditate easily. And study and think much better.

Since I kept my room clean and functional, it became a haven for everything you would expect I did in it. My room was used to play and joke with friends, study with them, listen to music, work, sleep, meditate—you name it. I found I was sleeping better, meditating deeper, being more creative and scoring better grades. Of course, meditation helped. But it's so much easier to get clean from the inside when you are clean from the outside.

Most importantly, I would look forward to going back to my room every evening after a full day of hard work and even harder play. I knew that this was my space to unwind, relax and rejuvenate.

So, even if you are living in a hostel or a really tiny house, what you will find in this chapter will go a long way in creating a space that is just perfect for you.

Let's begin!

First, get rid of anything in the bedroom that is not required for sleep. For example, I know many people who have a huge TV in their bedrooms. Sell it off. You don't want the light from that screen in the night, and you definitely don't want the mind agitation that will come from watching late-night TV shows or movies. Anything else you have in the bedroom that is not favourable for sleep, get rid of it.

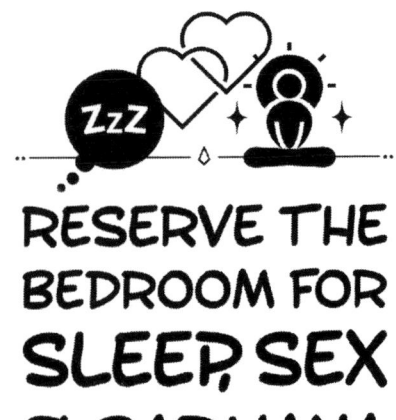

RESERVE THE BEDROOM FOR SLEEP, SEX & SADHANA

If your bedroom doubles up as your office, then clearly demarcate the areas for work and rest. Don't let your work stuff spill over into your space of rest.

Lights

Get really nice light fixtures. You want to have dimmable colour-changing lights so you can set the lighting to a dim warm yellow, or even a hazy red towards night. Being able to create some mood lighting in the bedroom is wonderful. I like to use lots of candles towards the late evening in my bedroom. Candles create a beautiful, warm, cozy ambience and somehow manage to induce deeper sleep. Remember to put out the candles before sleeping, or if you plan to leave your room for a long period of time.

While we are talking about lights, it's a great idea to **get dimmable lights for the bathroom** as well. If you do have to get up in the middle of the night to pee, the bright lights of most bathrooms can signal the brain that it's daytime and initiate your wake-up cycle. This is the reason why a lot of people have difficulty going back to sleep if they need to use the bathroom in the middle of the night.

While we are on the subject of lights, there is one more important consideration, which is often completely overlooked. Most people don't even know about it, and simply end up being victims of it. You see, most lights flicker, and that could cause problems. Let me explain.

Flicker

Try reading a book while someone rapidly turns the lights in your room on and off, on and off, on and off ... and you will understand the importance of using light fixtures with low flicker rates.

Any changes in the brightness of a light is called 'flicker'. Flicker is caused by the modulation of intensity of a light source.

Flicker is registered by your brain through your eyes. If you have ever been to a party with strobe lighting, you will notice

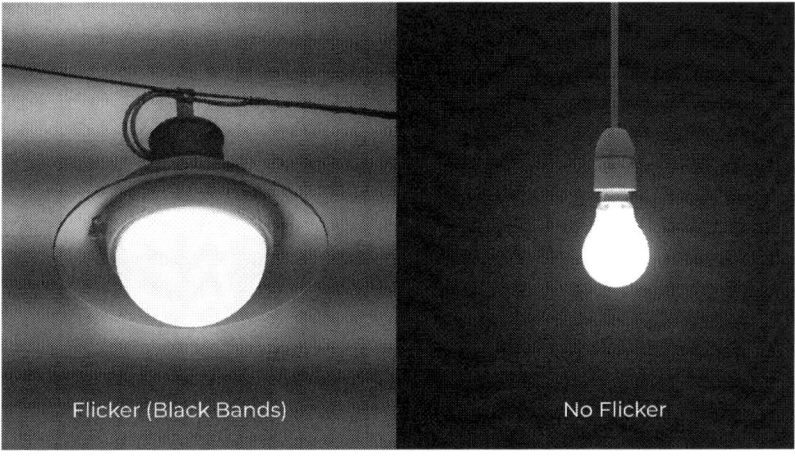

how for the first minute or two it looks quite amazing and all movement seems to slow down, feel somehow distorted, and look pretty cool.

Imagine now that the flashes of the strobe were made faster and faster so you could barely notice it. Your brain, would have to work hard to stitch these fast bursts and make things appear how they would in continuous lighting. This would make reading, writing or any task that required concentration disorienting and confusing. Your brain would be challenged each time you moved focus from one thing to another.

Lights with high flicker rates would hit our productivity and potentially create long-term health issues. Exposure to flicker when you are already feeling fatigued or sleep deprived can dramatically increase the detrimental effects of flicker.

Here are some health issues that can be caused through exposure to flicker, though the intensity would depend on personal photosensitivity. Children and young adults under the age of 20 are more at risk.

- Eye strain
- Headaches
- Neck pain and stiffness
- Chronic migraines
- Repetitive behaviors
- Nausea
- Vertigo
- Irritability
- Bad moods
- Photosensitive epilepsy
- Seizures
- Autism traits amplified
- Panic attacks

Almost any light that runs on Alternating Current (AC) from a plug point will have flicker. The power grid from where you get your electricity runs on 50 Hz (India) or 60 Hz (US), depending on which country you are in. Hertz or Hz is the number of cycles per second. This voltage change will cause the problem of flicker in light bulbs.

Incandescent lighting doesn't have this issue, because light is created by the heating of the filament in the bulb. As the voltage cycling is too fast for the filament to cool down and heat up again, it more or less stays heated and hence gives out light with extremely low flicker percentages.

LED lights are a different beast. They rapidly convert electrical energy to light. On AC this would mean extremely fast, barely noticeable strobe-like lighting. This is why an LED light has a driver that converts the AC to DC (Direct Current). Lights running on DC power will obviously be flicker free. Unfortunately, low quality drivers allow trickles from the AC line to leak through to the LED which would cause LEDs to flicker, even though they are technically running on DC.

It's quite easy to figure out if your LED light has a high flicker rate. Take a photo with your phone—a flare-like image means there is little to no flicker. Black, streaky lines mean there is high flicker and it is best that you get that lighting fixture changed. Note that when lights are dimmed, they will flicker more. Find a quick video about this on **www.booksbybnd.com/sys/media**.

The good news is that with high quality drivers in place, LED lighting can have low flicker rates, sometimes even better than an incandescent bulb that is not detrimental in any way for health or well-being.

There is a lot of complexity involved in actually measuring flicker, and a standard metric that has evolved is Stroboscopic Visibility Measure (SVM).

For the best lighting solutions, it is recommended that you use light fixtures with SVM < 1.3, for example, the Philips Base B22 9-Watt LED bulb in golden yellow.

Better than that? Natural lighting, of course. Open the windows, draw the curtains back and let the sun in!

It is best to **keep all your gadget charging stations outside your bedroom**. Their tiny lights can interfere with your sleep. And best to err on the side of caution, and keep whatever radiation these gadgets emanate as far away from yourself as possible. Towards late evening, turn off the Wi-Fi in your home. It might be a great idea to rope in your neighbours as well on this. I remember when I was up in Matheran and in Ranikhet, both beautiful hill stations with not-so-great Wi-Fi connectivity, I was sleeping much better than usual. These days, I ensure that I turn off the house Wi-Fi at night. We are lucky enough to be living in a stand-alone house with no other habitation around us for about 500 metres. Sleep quality definitely feels much better with the Wi-Fi off than when we leave it on.

Get blackout curtains for your windows. These can be hung behind your normal curtains so as not to spoil the aesthetics of your room. Drawing the curtains at night will eliminate the light coming in from outside, contributing to making your bedroom as dark as possible. To test if your bedroom is dark enough, draw the blackout curtains and switch off the lights. Then hold up your hands at an arm's length in front of your face. You shouldn't be able to see your fingers.

Air

Get a good air conditioner installed, especially if you live in a hot region. Your body needs to cool down to be able to sleep well. Hot weather can disrupt sleep. Ensure that you can shut off those teeny lights on the air conditioner. If you cannot, then some black duct tape will do the trick. You want the bedroom to be devoid of any light as you sleep.

As we sleep at night, we breathe out a lot of carbon dioxide (CO_2), which hangs around, especially in an air-conditioned room. If you feel a little heavy and tired when you wake up, even after a full 8 hours of deep, uninterrupted sleep, then CO_2 could be the culprit. The best way to handle this, and beautify your bedroom at the same time, is to get some plants. **The three best bedroom plants commonly available are the snake plant (or mother-in-law's tongue), the money plant and the areca palm.**

ARECA PALM

These plants convert CO_2 to oxygen at night and are fantastic to have in the bedroom. Check the appendix for instructions on how to care for these three plants. All are remarkably easy to maintain. Research says that you need seven of any one of these plants for each person sleeping in the room. But

SNAKE PLANT

I have seen really great results with even two or three in the room. Know that even two plants are better than none, though seven per person is best.

The other **must-have equipment in your bedroom is an air purifier**, especially if you live in a city. There are all sorts of pollutants and allergens in the air. These unseen particles can, over time, cause a lot of breathing issues, among other health problems. While you sleep, your immune system is up in arms against them, fighting to keep you healthy. With an air purifier doing a lot of the dirty work, your immune system gets a much-needed break to restore and rejuvenate itself during the night. Over a few weeks of usage, you will find yourself sleeping better and becoming healthier, and not falling sick often, as your immune system will regain its potency.

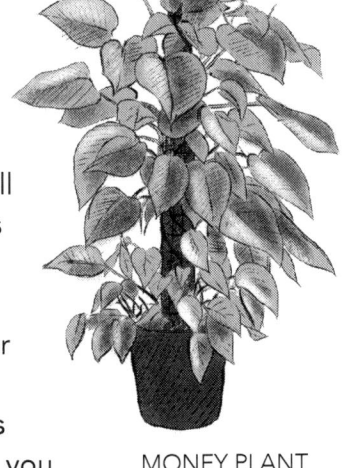

MONEY PLANT

Here are a few factors to consider before buying an air purifier:

- How much does it cost? Can you afford it? I have experimented with quite a few purifiers and the one that I finally settled on is called the IQ Air Health Pro 250. It costs a bomb, but is totally worth it. The amount of time and money saved by not being sick because of allergen and pollen is worth more than the Rs 1 lakh price tag on it. I have heard of people being completely free from chronic breathing problems like

asthma or allergic sneezing fits when they regularly sleep with an air purifier in their room.
- What are the running costs? Air purifier filters need to be replaced once a year or in two years, depending on your usage. Are those filters easily available? How expensive are they?
- How much noise does it make while running? If it makes too much noise, it may be difficult for some people to sleep. The IQ Air on low speeds hardly makes any noise, and the continuous white noise it does generate helps me sleep better.
- Does it have any LED lights? Can those be switched off or somehow muted? Even my super expensive air purifier didn't have any way to turn off the lights while it was on. I simply put 3–4 playing cards on the light panel and those tiny lights don't disturb the darkness in my bedroom at night.
- Does it have indicators to show that it is time to replace any of the filters? It is far better that the machine itself indicates the time for replacement rather than you playing some sort of a guessing game.
- Does it in any way emit ozone? Stay far away from these machines, as ozone is a known lung irritant, even if it says on the label that the ozone emission is well below the guidelines set out by the government.
- Does it have something called true High Efficiency Particulate Air (HEPA) filter technology? This is critical to have in an air purifier because this type of an air filter can theoretically remove at least 99.97% of dust, pollen, mould, bacteria, and any airborne particles of a size of 0.3 microns or more.

- Check the CADR number on the machine. CADR means Clean Air Delivery Rate and the higher this number is, the better the purifier. You will need higher CADR ratings for bigger rooms.
- Does the purifier have a big activated carbon filter? These absorb odour-causing molecules and cleanse the air of noxious smells that might come from various sources. Note that smaller carbon filters may not be able to do much; check with the manufacturer about the efficiency of the carbon filter in case you are thinking of buying a filter that has one.
- Don't buy filters with UV lights. To be effective, the UV light has to work on the air for a few minutes to a few hours, instead of the few seconds that the air will typically travel through it. Mostly UV light filters are a gimmick.
- Does your purifier have an energy star logo? Typically, an air purifier is mostly always on. A higher energy star rating means less electricity consumption.
- Does it have a good quality washable pre-filter? Better for the environment, cheaper on the pocket.
- Is it portable? Can it be rolled from room to room on wheels? Then you don't need to buy 4 purifiers for all 4 rooms of your home. Just 1 or 2 would be enough.
- Does it have a way of sucking in air from outside and purifying that? That would be a feature of a platinum standard air purifier, and if this is possible, even the CO_2 levels could potentially be controlled. Only a handful of air purifiers offer this feature.

Do your research before you get an air purifier. But make one a priority on your shopping list. Definitely don't buy one of those cheap ones on the market. They are worthless and a complete waste of money. A really good air purifier can make a tremendous difference to the quality of your life by enhancing your health and allowing you to rest deeper during sleep.

If you simply cannot afford an expensive air purifier then ensure you keep your space clean and as dust-free as possible. Don't keep books on open shelves, for example—they are dust magnets. Change your bedsheets as often as you can—at least once or twice a week. Vacuum your mattress, curtains and any seating you may have in your bedroom regularly. Though all this is by no means a replacement for a good air purifier, it may help.

Sound

Strangely, a perfectly quiet room may actually hinder your sleep. Of course, an extremely noisy room would make it almost impossible for most people to fall asleep in. I have to tell you a story about this …

I was teaching an Art of Living course in Asia's biggest slum, Dharavi in Mumbai. Many attending the course were people who lived literally day-to-day, wretchedly poor. If the wage earner didn't get work for the day, the family wouldn't be able to eat that night. Our courses there were a huge hit. We taught them Yoga, Pranayama and Meditation and more than 90% of those who attended gave up on their vices. Their quality of life improved. With the collective help of our volunteer group in Mumbai and the people who had done the courses in Dharavi, we cleaned up a big area that was designated to be a garden, but was used as a dump. More than 40 truckloads of garbage later, we had a nice little garden, with a lawn, some ashoka trees and a small shed which they made into a gym for the local boys to come and exercise in.

One old, old man was quite active and would contribute a lot in all our efforts, and we became pretty pally with him. He would wear tattered clothes and had a completely unkempt appearance, but he was quite resourceful. He would always know who we should speak to, to make things happen.

One evening we were chatting with him, and I mentioned that we were looking for a place to teach courses in the Hiranadani Gardens in Powai—an exclusive upmarket area where houses cost crores of rupees. He casually remarked that he had a 5-bedroom house there and we could use it if we wanted to.

We were aghast. He had a humungous penthouse in one of Mumbai's finest housing complexes and he still lived in Dharavi?!

He smiled and said, 'I just can't sleep in that house. If there is no noise and no smell, no sleep comes. I have grown up here and I will die here. You use the house for your courses. All of you are doing such great work. It will be my privilege to help you.'

Humans indeed are creatures of habit and habitat.

It is you who needs to be comfortable with the sound levels in your bedroom. Many cannot sleep in a perfectly quiet room. Some people even use a white noise machine because it helps them sleep better. For me, the gentle purring noise from my AC and air purifier is enough to lull me into comfortable slumber. I must admit that after spending almost fifteen years in the quiet peace of the Art of Living ashram in rural Bangalore, I find it difficult to sleep with the noise, hustle and bustle of any big city. When I travel for courses, and I do that a lot, I long for my own room, my own bed, my own blanket and my own pillows.

Which brings us to the bed itself.

The Bed

The centerpiece of the story. This is where all the action … I mean the inaction happens.

For your bed, the cheapest option would be to go back to the basics. Don't listen to all that advertising about all those foamy, soft, space-age type mattresses. Go to your trusty gadda-wala in the local market, and get him to make you a traditional cotton mattress with the best possible organic cotton used for stuffing. The stuffing makes or breaks the mattress, so insist on really good material. The mattress shouldn't be soft and floppy. It should be firm and comfortable. I would recommend a thickness of about 2 inches.

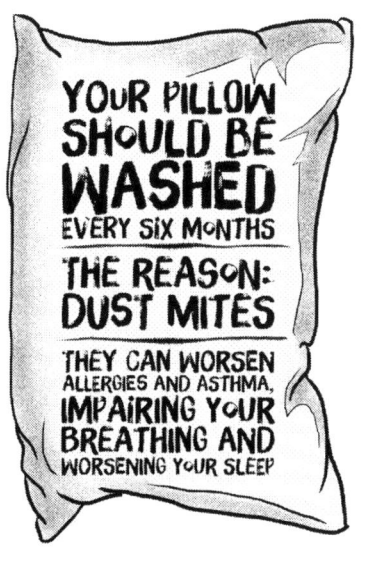

By sheer chance, we stumbled upon mattresses made by PEPS India. These are fairly expensive mattresses and frankly, we were quite sceptical about them helping make our sleep better. We had already spent crazy amounts of money trying all sorts of mattresses, and would always keep coming back to the basic cotton gadda. However, the owner of PEPS India turned out to be the cousin of a dear friend, and she introduced us to him. Shankarram truly believes his products are world-class and is utterly passionate about great sleep—just like us. He insisted that we try out his mattresses and quite reluctantly, we said yes.

We are sooooo glad we did.

His mattresses are absolutely brilliant. They are firm, yet comfortable and don't mess with your spine and back as you sleep. Our sleep quality has definitely improved and we have no hesitation in recommending PEPS India mattresses. They used only the best quality of material to make their mattresses and it shows. The ones we have used and loved are Organica, SpineGuard and Restonic. Even their SpringKoil is pretty good, but that would be a second choice for us.

As a cheap option, your pillows can be made by your local gadda-wala—with a thickness of about the width of your shoulder. The only pillow I liked from PEPS India was their Neck Guard Memory Molded Pillow—Contour. We tried some of their other pillows but I personally didn't find them as nice as the Memory Molded Contour pillow. I guess pillows are a personal choice, and you should experiment with a few to see which ones you find most comfortable. You know you have a great pillow when you don't wake up with neck pain.

I have found these to be the absolute best solution for having great sleep and a healthy spine. All those other fancy soft mattresses sold in the name of comfort only compromise your back, creating all sorts of painful kinks and make osteopaths and craniosacral therapists rich.

Linen

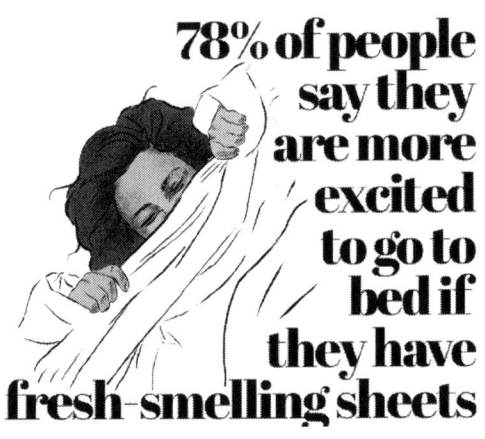

Invest in getting the softest, highest thread count cotton or bamboo silk bedsheets and pillow covers that you possibly can. The material should make you feel like you are sleeping on a cloud. Get luxurious warm blankets that you know you will love to cocoon yourself in. Splurge on the bed linen and get the finest you can afford.

Twice or thrice a week vacuum all the mattresses, pillows, blankets and sheets. You will be truly aghast at the amount of dust your machine will suck up. Of course, I don't need to tell you that it's a great idea to change all the linen on a regular basis.

Paint the bedroom walls in light shades—a soothing beige is best according to me. Avoid blatant colours like fire engine red, for example. Use muted colours, or just pale soft whites. Similarly, use curtains with understated designs—nothing that will stand out, yet will add to the beauty of the room with muted elegance.

Do all you can to create a space that invites you to relax and unwind. Once the stage is set, your romance with sleep will blossom as she whisks you away into her beguiling embrace, bestowing you with the rest that you crave for and deserve at the end of each day.

Good Night!

The Winding Down Ritual

It's 5 p.m. and you know it's time for your exercise. You wind up whatever you are doing, and get ready. You pack your shoes, socks, gym clothes and gloves, get your bottle of water, eat an orange, and then head to the gym to exercise.

Once you are at the gym, you get into proper gym attire. Have a swig of water. Then do some warm ups before you get into your exercise routine.

Right?

If you are going out to dinner with someone special, the preparation is even more detailed. Shower, shave (or wax), cologne, smart clothes, hair styled properly, good shoes … You would take a good 30 minutes to an hour to get yourself ready for that date.

Right?

You've got a few good friends coming home for a Sunday lunch. Your prep for that might start the day before. Get the home clean, figure out a menu, decide on the music playlist, think about which movie to watch or which board game to play, get the food cooked, get into good clothes …

Right?

You have an important presentation to make at your office. You might spend a week or more getting the data in place. Then a few days making the slide deck and getting all your notes together. At least a few hours on the aesthetic of how everything is looking and if the flow of the presentation works. Possibly doing a few mock presentations to stay within the time limit allotted to you.

On the day of the event, you will groom yourself to look and feel your best. Show up early and make sure all the technology works. All of us have done all this and more, many, many times in life.

Right?

There is one crucial ingredient that will contribute significantly to your success in all these situations. And that ingredient is enough good quality sleep. Without sleep, your muscles will not grow, however much you exercise, and food will not get digested properly. Delete sleep and you lose your intelligence and charm. And you age faster.

For some activities, people spend days, weeks, even years getting ready. In India, I have heard that prepping for the IIT entrance exam starts seven to eight years in advance (a completely stupid thing to do, in my opinion). Yet, the parents of these children (and the children themselves) give hardly an iota of importance to sleep. That regular sleeping habits make you smarter is an established scientific fact utterly ignored by most people.

Let me repeat this—enough good quality sleep makes you younger, smarter, sexier and healthier. Every single organ and system of the body is positively impacted by proper sleep.

Just as you prep to go to the gym and have a great workout, or spend time getting ready for a hot date, or work for an exam, a presentation or an interview, you need to give time to prep to have a great night's sleep. Most people's prep for sleep consists of flopping into bed, not even bothering to get out of their daytime clothes, and going to sleep. Even if they get their 8 hours of sleep, the quality will be compromised. This chapter is all about 'Sleep Hygiene'—

creating a winding-down ritual for yourself so that you are guaranteed the best possible sleep quality ever.

We have seen in an earlier chapter that the onset of sleep is created by two independent systems in the body. The sleep drive and the circadian rhythm. When these two systems peak together, a fantastic window of opportunity is created to go to sleep. Sleep hygiene is ensuring that both these systems are optimised.

My five non-negotiable steps for sleep hygiene:
1. No caffeine after 2 p.m. and not more than 2 cups of coffee or tea in a day. Remember that caffeine is 10x more potent than white light at sleep disruption.
2. Limited or no exposure to white and blue light three hours before bedtime. For every hour of white light exposure, your melatonin secretion is pushed forward by about half an hour. Please change all light fittings in your home to warm yellow. Install the white light blocking apps on all your screens.
3. Dinner at least three to four hours before bedtime. A more or less empty stomach when you sleep means that the energy of the body during sleep is used for repairing and rejuvenating the body instead of digesting food.
4. Stop the usage of electronic screens—phones, tablets, computers, TVs, etc., an hour before bedtime. It gives your mind time to unwind.
5. A completely dark, comfortable and cool bedroom. Even the smallest of lights in a darkened room can intrude on your sleep. The tiny green light of an air conditioner or the blinking light of your computer that is charging can stop you from resting deeply. Sleep science has shown that we sleep deeper and tend not to awaken during the night when the bedroom is comfortably cooled—any temperature between 18 to 24 degrees Celsius.

Get these five in place and you are more than 70% there.

Assuming you have the five points above in place and you don't want to settle for anything other than 7-star quality sleep (like I do), more or less in chronological order, follow these steps:

Watch the sunset. Seeing the whites and blues of the day transform into the yellows, pinks and oranges of the evening and finally fading into the darkness of the night sends a powerful cue to the brain and the circadian rhythm to begin the prep for sleep.

Decide your bedtime. What time are you going to get into bed to sleep each night—even on weekends? As we saw in the chapter 'Falling Asleep', maintaining a standard bedtime and wake up time helps the circadian rhythm to enhance itself. Set an alarm to go off 2 to 3 hours before your chosen bedtime to signal the start of your winding down routine.

As soon as your alarm goes off, give yourself 30-40 minutes of finishing off with screens. Deal with whatever social media, WhatsApp, messages and emails need to be dealt with. Have the alarm go off again after 40 minutes and shut down your screens as soon as it goes off. This, perhaps, is the hardest thing to do. There is always one more message, one more cute video, one more funny post to read. All that can wait. You wouldn't spend any time on any of that if you were getting ready to go on a hot date, would you?

If you are not a social media person, then take this time to play a relaxing board game with your family. Mumbai Connection, the board game we made, is highly recommended!

Shut down those screens. Now.
Another 20-30 minutes to finish household chores and get things ready for tomorrow. Do those dishes, prep the veggies, clear out the garbage, feed the cat, iron and lay out the clothes you are going to wear the next day, make your bed ... **Finish the tasks of the day.**

Drink a glass of water. Avoid drinking water too close to bedtime. It could make you want to get up to pee in the night.

After this, you don't need that alarm any more.

Dim the lights in your bedroom. Perhaps light a few candles. Turn on the air conditioning if required, to cool your bedroom down to whatever is a comfortable temperature for you, between 18 and 24 degrees Celsius.

Finish all personal hygiene like brushing your teeth, etc. **Take a hot shower**, preferably in candlelight or using very dim lighting in the bathroom. The hot water will force the blood to your skin's surface and bring down your core body temperature. For sleep to be deep, your core body temperature needs to fall by a few degrees. The hot water shower will do that for you. It would be a great idea to pamper your skin at this point—especially your face. Use a good high quality delicate facial cleanser to cleanse your face. Pat dry. Spritz with really good rose water and let it dry. Then depending on your skin type apply a good moisturiser, especially where your face has a tendency to form wrinkles. Watch our video on how we do this super relaxing little routine on **www.booksbybnd.com/sys/media.**

For the rest of your body, a little cream or oil lovingly rubbed in feels just fantastic.

Get into clean, loose, comfortable nightclothes. There are some sleep experts who say sleeping naked is best, but if that is not your cup of tea, get the softest, most luxurious, most comfortable nightwear you can get and wear that. Changing into nightclothes is another powerful signal to the body that you are ready for sleep. Do not sleep in your day clothes, or unwashed clothes from the night before. Use fresh clothes each night for sleep.

Read the Shopping Guide in the Appendix to know more about the products we use to get ready for sleep.

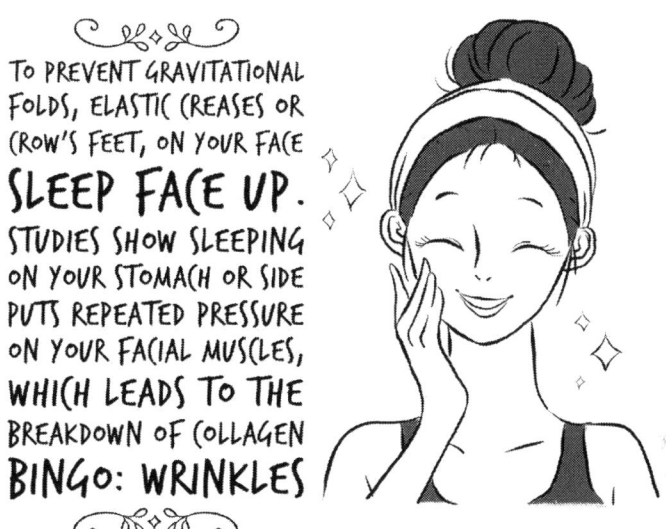

To prevent gravitational folds, elastic creases or crow's feet, on your face **SLEEP FACE UP.** Studies show sleeping on your stomach or side puts repeated pressure on your facial muscles, which leads to the breakdown of collagen **BINGO: WRINKLES**

Do some light stretches for a few minutes. Remember not to overdo this at all. Exercise releases cortisol which is a 'wake up' hormone. Any sort of vigourous physical activity after 7 p.m. will interfere with your sleep. The stretching simply releases tight muscles and allows you deeper rest through the night. See the video on 'Yoga for Great Sleep', for our recommended set of stretches on **www.booksbybnd.com/sys/media.**

Now you have some options; choose to do as many of them you wish to:

- Read a few pages of a book—something pleasant like this book—nothing violent please.
- Chit-chat a bit (not on the phone; screen time is over—only with whoever happens to be there with you).
- A small cup of hot milk, unsweetened and unflavoured, or malt milk or turmeric pepper milk with a drop of ghee are fantastic for great sleep.

- Vegans can have a cup of herbal tea. Chamomile tea is universally accepted as a great sleep inducer. Other teas include lavender, valerian root, spearmint and passionflower and combinations of the above. Do not sweeten the tea and make sure it is decaffeinated. Otherwise it will defeat the purpose of having that tea.
- Listen to some chanting. I love the Devi Kavacham by Bhanumati Narasimhan.
- Read a page or two of the *Bhagavad Gita* or the *Yoga Vasishtha*.
- Do some journaling. I like to write out 5 things I am grateful for today, with the challenge that I never repeat anything I have already written. There are quite a few studies that say that this activity, when done over a few months without a break, physically alters the brain which, in turn, transforms your attitude towards life.
- If there is anything that you have to remember to do, write that out. Keep one place where you write this—so you always know where to find it. This allows the brain to relax and not try to 'remember' things that need to be done. This minimises mind activity when you get into bed, making it so much easier to quickly drift off to sleep.

Engage yourself in any relaxing activity, that pleases your mind. Do not watch the news, some TV serial, movie or senseless debate. Anyways by now you are off all screens. At this point, we don't want to agitate anything within us.

Think of one or two things (not more) that you wish to accomplish the next day and write these out in brief. Doing this prompts your brain to seek solutions or ideas during REM sleep. It taps into the 'smart' part of your brain. You will invariably wake up with a brilliant idea or an obvious solution that you somehow had never thought of before.

Switch off all lights, put out the candles and completely darken your bedroom.
Get into bed.
Sit and stare in the darkness for about 10 minutes. This can help improve your eyesight. 80% of the 'seeing' apparatus of our eyes is geared towards darkness, and we hardly use it.
Do some alternate nostril breathing—Nadi Shodhan Pranayama as it is called. See the alternate nostril breathing video for how to do this on **www.booksbybnd.com/sys/media.** A few minutes of this type of breathing will balance your body and you will get great sleep. Exhalation should be longer than inhalation. If you are breathing in for 4 counts, hold for 4 counts and exhale for 8 counts. Hold the exhalation for 2 counts.
Lie on your back. Cover yourself up with your blanket …
Do the Power Yoga Nidra—squeezing and relaxing each muscle group at a time will release soreness and tension throughout the body. See the Power Yoga Nidra video for instructions for doing this.
There is this one last thing I personally do each night. **The Belly Rub.** There was a Japanese Zen monk, almost a hundred years old, who had visited our ashram in Bangalore. He was a healer and looked not more than 60 or 65. He was remarkably fit and supple. When we asked him for one thing we could do to age as gracefully as he had, he said, 'Rub your belly with the right hand, clockwise around the belly button, in fairly big circles, exactly 200 times just before going to sleep. Not 199. Not 201. 200. He said do this from now on for the rest of your life. So I do it. And maybe you should too.
Smile, feel grateful that you had one more day on this beautiful planet of ours.

As she would tuck me into bed, my mother used to say in a singsong voice:

Good Night
Sleep tight
Keep you safe from harm
Always.

And *savaarsavaar ma hasta ramta uthi jajo*, which meant may you wake up smiling, laughing and in a playful mood.

My favourite mantra to chant just before sleeping is:
*Kaayena Vaacha Manasendriyairva
Budhyaatmanaava Prakrati Swabhaavaat
Karomi Yadyat Sakalam Parasmai
Naaraayanaayeti Samarpayaami
Om Shanti, Shanti, Shantihi*

I feel this is the ultimate little prayer to chant just before sleep. Here is what it means:
Through my body, or my speech, my thoughts and feelings, or my senses

कायेन वाचा मनसेन्द्रियैर्वा ।
बुद्ध्यात्मना वा प्रकृतेः स्वभावात् ।
करोमि यद्यत्सकलं परस्मै ।
नारायणायेति समर्पयामि ॥
ॐ शान्तिः शान्तिः शान्तिः

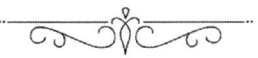

Through my intellect, or my consciousness, or because of my very nature,

Whatever I have done so far (or has happened because of me),

I offer it all to you, Lord Narayana.

May there be peace in my body and mind, peace in the environment and peace in all the subtle and invisible realms.

You can listen to this little chant and some other soothing night-time chants in **www.booksbybnd.com/sys/media.**

Create a winding down ritual for yourself. Every night, go through each step faithfully. As you continue to do the ritual night after night, you are sending powerful signals to your brain to allow the magic of sleep to work its wonders on you.

Sweet Dreams …

Good Night!

P.S.: There are a few more things to do for great sleep, but those involve waking up—check out the next chapter!

The Art of Waking Up

While you were sleeping, our planet rotated around its axis at approximately 1670 km/hr to bring you back to daylight—and a brand-new day!

Hopefully, by now, you have a fantastic winding down ritual in place that you practice every night, to get deeply restful sleep. You awaken naturally, feeling rejuvenated and relaxed, and excited about the new day ahead.

Unfortunately, too many people are viciously roused awake by their alarm clocks. They will usually hit the snooze button a few times and are rudely jolted into wakefulness each time, compounding the already malefic effect of the alarm. Habitually woken up by an alarm clock, however sweet-sounding, has been shown to increase risk of hypertension, cardiac issues and even stroke.

Then they sleepily tumble out of bed and shamble into their bathroom, finish their morning bathroom routine and find themselves in the kitchen, making some hot beverage that they feel will actually wake them up and get them ready to face the day. They are always in a hurry and reach their place of work already feeling tired—and it's not even mid-morning.

If this even remotely resembles your morning routine, stop doing this to yourself. There is an art to waking up, and it begins with getting an 8-hour sleep opportunity each night. Ensure you have a clear 8 hours to sleep and awaken naturally without the need of an alarm clock. We use the alarm clock in a different way from the rest of the world—to set the time to begin our winding down ritual.

As you wake up, there will be a few precious moments of transcendence—where you are neither asleep nor quite awake. Sleep is gently giving way to wakefulness. Enjoy this space. As you journey towards full wakefulness, you could cuddle with the person in bed with you. This raises the levels of oxytocin and serotonin in your system, putting you in a great mood that will last throughout the day. Sleep experts say that this is perhaps the best time to have sex.

When you are fully awake, don't lounge around in bed. Even though the bed is warm and comfortable and the room is deliciously cool and the feeling of 'just 5 minutes more' is overwhelming, get out of bed to begin your day. You can spend 5 minutes in bed just before jumping out. In those 5 minutes, become aware of all the parts of your body that are feeling good, strong and healthy. Too often our attention is drawn to the aches and pains. Acknowledge those, but spend some time appreciating the rest of the body that is doing well. This little act of awareness will spread more and more health in your system, and, over time, you will find you wake up with far less pain and brain fog than you used to.

Finish your morning routine in the bathroom, and come back and make your bed. Making your bed first thing in the morning takes less than 5 minutes, but it gives you a delightful squirt of dopamine—a powerful feel-good hormone, setting your motivation levels high for the day.

You lose approximately a litre of water through your breath every night as you sleep. Hydrate yourself by drinking 2 glasses of water right away—about ½ a litre of water is great for everyone. Add in a lime shot—the juice of one lime and 2-3 tablespoons of warm water to alkalise your system—a truly great way to start the day.

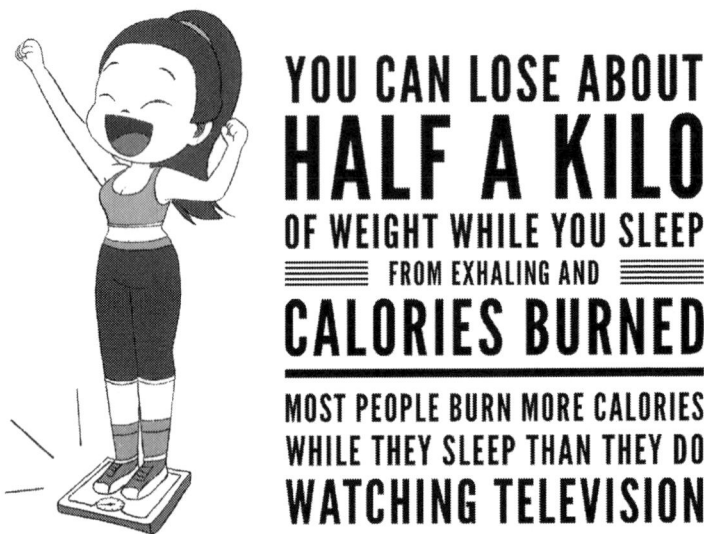

If you are an early riser, this would be a great time to meditate. I have practised the techniques taught through Sri Sri Ravi Shankar's Art of Living for almost three decades and wholeheartedly recommend that you learn and practice them. Meditation at this time can totally relax you, clear up brain fog and get you energised for the rest of the day. Visit **www.inergyworld.com** for the schedules of courses taught by Dinesh, me and our team and **www.artofliving.org** for more about the organisation.

Catch half an hour of morning sunlight. Go for a nice long walk, and as we saw in an earlier chapter, remember NOT to wear sunglasses. Your brain gets cues for day and night from the eyes. Wear sunglasses and even at midday, your brain will register that you are in the dark.

The Earth–Body Connection

When you go for your morning walk, spend as much time as you can walking barefoot on the earth. This 'grounds' you. You can walk barefoot on grass, or on the beach or on mud—not on asphalt. It's even better if the surface is a little wet. Even swimming in a river, a lake or an ocean will do the trick.

There are many scientific studies about the tremendous benefits of grounding—it minimises, and in many cases, even eliminates inflammation in the body.

The white blood cells in our body naturally produce oxidative loads, popularly called free radicals, to fight off infections and protect sites of injury. On the molecular battlefields of our bodies, white blood cells fight infection by unloading free radicals, which have a lust for electrons. They kill the intruders by stripping them off their electrons, thus stabilising themselves.

This process works brilliantly. Except that our white blood cells can be quite enthusiastic in their zeal to protect us, and many times unload considerably more free radicals than required. This is a problem. Once the intruders have been dealt with, these free radicals turn on healthy tissue in the vicinity and strip that of its electrons, and end up creating an injury.

The immune system registers the injury and even more white blood cells gather in their droves to nullify the damage, but end up causing even more damage. This vicious circle is what is called an inflammatory response.

Besides this, the electromagnetic field generated by any plugged-in electronic equipment will create a massive buildup of free radicals in our system if you happen to be sufficiently near it. Just typing stuff out on your laptop (which is plugged in) or talking or texting on a mobile phone that is charging is enough to stockpile the free radicals.

Look around and see how many pieces of electronic gadgetry surround you right now. All this adds up to the problem of excess free radicals and compounds the woes of our body as it fights a desperate battle with itself, trying to protect itself.

Inflammation robs you of your vitality and health and causes almost all the so-called lifestyle diseases. Chronic pain and stiffness, arthritis, allergies, asthma, autoimmune diseases, coeliac disease, IBS and even certain cancers are directly related to inflammation. The effects of these terrible diseases can be reduced or even eliminated if the inflammation is neutralised. A new term was used by the person who 'discovered' grounding—Clinton Ober—inflammageing.

Enter the antioxidants.

Antioxidants have extra electrons and hence can satisfy and stabilise the free radicals and prevent them from inflicting havoc on the body. People do all sorts of things to get their antioxidants—from popping pills to eating healthy antioxidant-rich food.

They have not realised something very basic …

Lightning strikes the surface of the Earth almost 100 times a second—that's about 8 million times a day or 3 billion times a year, suffusing the surface with—you guessed it—electrons!

The Earth has an almost infinite supply of the negatively charged electrons that we so badly need in our bodies. The amazing thing is that all we need to do to access the electron-rich supply of the Earth is simply touch it with our bare skin. Which as a species we had been doing for millions of years, throughout evolution. Until Charles Goodyear created rubber in 1839. Which soon led to the invention of shoes with rubber soles. Which all of us wear through the day. Which isolate and insulate us from the electron-rich surface of the Earth. It is ironical that we live on the Earth and yet are so completely disconnected from it.

Hello inflammation!

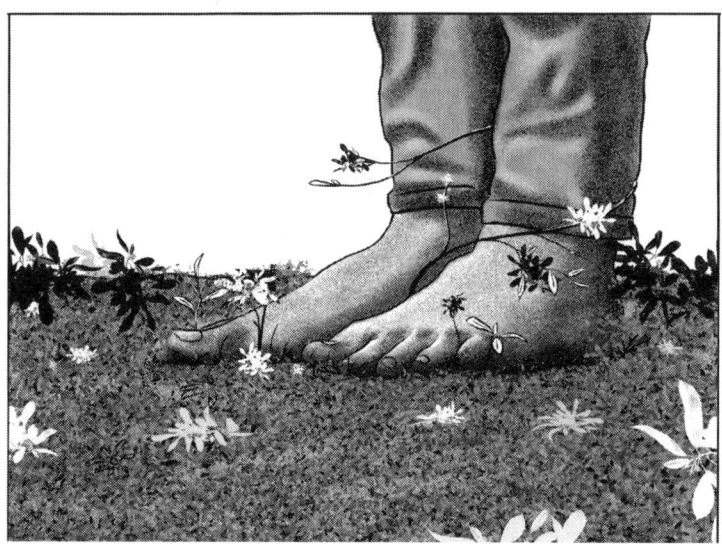

Clinton Ober's insight was that the Earth itself is the biggest antioxidant 'pill'—and all we need is to get our bare skin in contact with the Earth, and the problem of inflammation, and therefore a myriad of unpleasant health conditions, are sorted. When our bare skin touches the Earth's surface, electrons surge through our body and neutralise any free radicals that might be present.

Grounding may be the simplest way to increase antioxidants in the body and reduce or eliminate the destructive action of the free radicals. Over time, this translates to rapid reduction in pain and swelling all over the body. Your cortisol levels will drop and you will experience less stress. Of course, you will sleep deeper and therefore function better. You need between half an hour to 2 hours of grounding each day, through the day. The more hours you ground yourself daily, the better.

There is an entire range of grounding products available. Unfortunately, most of these products are US or Europe based, and exorbitantly expensive to buy in India. As awareness about the fabulous benefits of grounding become more well known, I am sure these simple, effective products will soon be available in India as well. In fact, just before this book went to press, I found a small Indian company that makes grounding mats and imports grounding sheets. I reached out to them, and they have promised to bring in more grounding products over the next year or two. Their website is **www.groundingindia.com.** You can read more about them in the Shopping Guide in the Appendix. Support them by buying your grounding mat and sheets from them.

A grounding bedsheet is typically made of high quality cotton which is interwoven with extremely thin silver wires. When you sleep on this, you stay grounded the entire night. While a grounding mat is simple to make at home—I am using the mat Dinesh and I made as I type this out, you will need to buy a grounding bedsheet. Grounding products ensure that even when you are not outside, you still continue to remain grounded and reap the resulting benefits. Check out my video on grounding and how to make your own grounding mat from **www.booksbybnd.com/sys/media** and just in case you feel it's too much trouble to make, or you are simply feeling lazy about it, order your mat from **www.groundingindia.com.**

Dinesh and I have been routinely grounding ourselves for a while now and for something that is so supremely simple to do, the quality of life enhancements have been nothing short of spectacular. In particular, the aches and pains I used to have when I would wake up in the morning have reduced by more than 70%. I have definitely become much more flexible as well.

I have heard stories of people who couldn't even move because of terrible arthritic pain. Who couldn't even go to the toilet without help. They have been able to get up and walk around with minimal pain after just a week of grounding for more than 3-4 hours each day.

Don't make the costly mistake of severing the connection of your body to our lovely planet. There is a reason that around the world, cultures from time immemorial have referred to our planet as Mother Earth. The Earth itself will rid you of so many health issues, if you will only let it.

Breakfast

Once you are back home, treat yourself to a green smoothie—refer to the recipe in the chapter 'Adding by Subtracting'. Just a month of green smoothies coupled with your barefoot morning walk will considerably improve your sense of overall wellbeing. The green smoothie will flood your system will all sorts of wonderful vitamins and minerals and give a fantastic kickstart to various systems of your body.

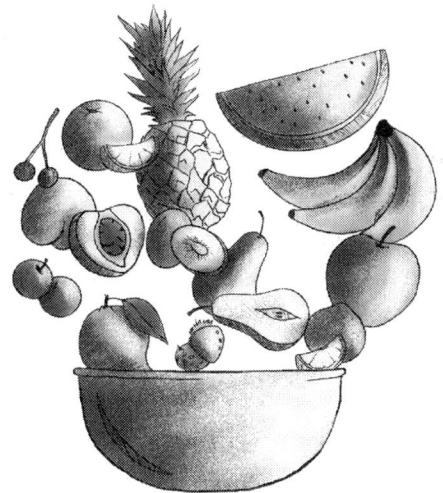

You could have a big bowl of fruits of different colours next. Pause for about 15-20 minutes after this before you have your usual cooked breakfast. Many people report that after the smoothie and the fruits they don't want to eat anything else—that is perfectly fine too.

Intermittent fasting—fasting for 14 hours or more each day—is a great idea, with innumerable health benefits. If your dinner was at 7 or even 8 p.m., then have your smoothie at around 10 a.m.

You had a candle-lit hot shower at night. In the morning, end your shower with alternate bursts of hot and cold water—you should especially splash the cold water on your forehead. 10 to 15 seconds of hot water, followed by 20 to 30 seconds of cold water—repeat at least 5 times. This will help you shed stubborn fat when you exercise. Besides, it feels amazingly invigorating.

Notice that, so far, I have not mentioned anything about social media, TV, phone messages, newspapers, etc. Devote the precious time early in the morning to thinking about what it is you truly want to manifest in your life and consequently, what steps you need to take to get it. Read the chapter 'Pizza of Life' in this book and take this time to complete the recommended processes. This is perhaps the best time in the day to do it.

Hint: Checking messages, answering emails, watching the news and surfing Facebook and Instagram will not in any way contribute to turning your dream to reality. Dinesh and I do a lot of our thinking during our morning walks. Many ideas, including the idea for this book, came from pleasant conversations we have while we walk, ground and take in the morning sun.

If you are a coffee or tea person, have your hot beverage at around 11 a.m. to get the full effect of the caffeine. This will help you be a little more productive in the afternoon. Though, if you ask me, around 2 p.m. is a great time to catch a quick nap of 20-30 minutes to reset the Sleep Drive and keep you fresh and alert till late evening.

Here is a summary of the Art of Waking Up:

1. Wake up naturally, without an alarm
2. Wake up at more or less the same time each day, even on weekends
3. Once awake, cuddle or get out of bed right away—don't give in to the 'just 5 more minutes' syndrome
4. Bathroom stuff and make your bed
5. Lime shot + 2 glasses of water
6. Meditate
7. Walk and ground for at least 30 minutes
8. Green smoothie and fruits, preferably after 10 a.m.
9. End your bath with a hot and cold shower
10. Drink your hot beverage only after 11 a.m.

You can move some stuff around. There are many people I know who prefer to meditate towards evening. Others like to meditate after their walk instead of before. Some like to take their bath as soon as they are out of their beds. I will leave all this shuffling to you.

Use the morning to plan and action your big life goals—things that truly matter to you. Don't fritter away this precious time by answering emails and messages, or surfing the net.

You might think that this is a long list of things to do and feel quite sure you have no time to do all of it, or even half of it. You have kids to send to school, you have that long commute to work, you have food to cook …

Simply deciding that you will do this will allow you to make time for it. And if you have to, at least in the beginning steal time and make it happen. This is the 20% that super optimises the rest of the 80%. Do this set and you will find yourself doing other things much more efficiently and creatively. You will be healthier, feel younger and become a far more pleasant person to be with.

Have a lovely day ahead …

Good Morning!

Guess?

Mankind thru' the ages is still quite unsure,
What womenkind want, or how they charm 'n lure!
But both kind should be clear what dangers lurk,
And how cruel life can get, when Her charms won't work.

Does She exist as particles, or does She come in waves,
Wonder if we are the masters, or simply Her slaves?!
Should we wrack our brains to understand Her,
Or Just surrender to Her power
Using Her to gain success, grow fitter 'n wiser?!

Our brain and spinal cord are floating in sparkly magic fluid,
That CSF has concoctions befitting the workings of a druid.
The balanced ebb and flow of this fluidy light,
Turns on a soothing, soporific effect all night.

Daily being busy; caught up with matters important or not,
Floods our brain with villainous toxins, and thickens the plot,
Nightly, our bodies and brain tissues relax, and create extra space
Helping flush toxic chemicals, and unwanted memories erase.

Guess?

She can come in cycles, each an hour and a half,
With all Her finer details, She generates a complicated graph.
Five of these cycles are needed and necessary,
To enjoy all Her benefits—cake, topping and cherry.

Neither at home, nor at medical school are we taught,
How keenly Her charms should be sought.
She is the best builder of muscle,
In addition, burning fat She does as a cool side hustle.

Many may know muscle fibres breakdown during exercise,
Nutrition and growth hormones nightly, make them resize.
And burn fat the body does only when it feels free of stress,
By now, you should know who can relieve it, c'mon—take an educated guess!

— Dinesh Ghodke

Sleep and the Three Vital Energies

The ancient Indian medical system of Ayurveda says that everything, including us, is made up of five primordial elements—Space, Air, Fire, Water and Earth. These elements combine with each other to form the three 'Vital Energies' or Doshas that quite uniquely create our basic nature.

Vata, the first, is formed by the combination of space and air. Vata is movement, and is responsible for all the movement that happens in and with our bodies. The movement of your eyeballs as you read this sentence, the flow of blood in your arteries and veins, the breath going in and out of your nostrils, you getting up to answer the doorbell—any and all movement is governed by Vata. A Vata person is usually quick and creative.

Think of air and space—when air is benign, it's like a gentle breeze, soothing and calming. When you have enough space, you feel expanded and rested. This is Vata behaving itself. Storms of emotions, feelings of being caged, impairment in movement of any sort and dryness is Vata derangement. Disturbed Vata can mean moodiness, a distracted mind, anxiety issues and bad sleep.

Pitta, the second, is the interaction between fire and water. Pitta regulates metabolism in the body. Pitta digests and assimilates. Pitta ensures that you get nourishment from the food you eat. Pitta people are typically determined, exhibit strong leadership qualities, are remarkably intelligent and are quick learners.

Fire will give warmth. Fire is the catalyst for life. Fire brings a sense of security. Fire is bright. Water flows and is adaptable. The feelings of cordiality, being safe and being healthy are all indications of Pitta in equilibrium. A glow on your face, keenness of intellect, the ability to be agile and adapt to situations are all gifts of Pitta. Think of a raging fire, though, and its ability to devastate, and you will get an inkling of Pitta being out of whack. Anger and agitation in the mind, ulcers, inflammation, acidity or any sort of burning disease are all warnings that your Pitta needs attention. Imbalances in Pitta can make you impatient, create personal conflicts, bring on rage, resentment and mood swings.

Kapha, the third, is created through earth and water. Kapha is all about strength, stamina, structure and stability. Kapha is grounding in nature. Kapha lubricates, hydrates and keeps things in the body moving fluidly. Kapha is involved in the immune response of the body. Kapha people are empathetic, trusting and caring, wise and mature, calm and happy by nature.

The Earth is all-accepting in nature. She is the platform on which life happens. Proper kapha means that your bodily structure will be stable and strong. You will be thoughtful, calm and steady in your approach to life. A Kapha person can be stubborn as well, and when provoked beyond their limits, becomes quite dangerous. Think earthquakes—they rarely happen, but when they do, they cause untold misery and suffering. All growth and structure-related bodily issues, as well as laziness and lethargy in the mind, are the effect of a disturbance in Kapha. Sluggishness, gaining weight rather quickly, depression and a tendency to oversleep are all indications of Kapha disruption.

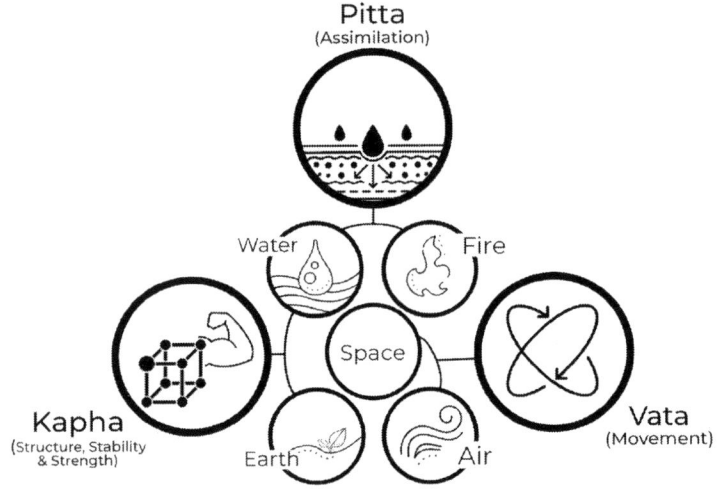

Good health, according to Ayurveda, is all about ensuring that these three vital energies are in balance. There are innumerable herbs, treatments and procedures to help create this balance—but it all finally boils down to creating a lifestyle that matches and balances your particular combination of the three doshas. This happens through the practice of yoga and meditation, combined with proper sleep and good healthy food.

The great sages and seers of ancient India, tens of thousands of years ago, talked about the aspects of Ayurveda in their various texts. Proper sleep is considered one of the main pillars of health in Ayurveda. Since this is a book about sleep, here is a quick snapshot of what they had to say about sleep. It is amazingly similar to what sleep science, after decades of research, and spending billions of dollars, is saying today.

Enough good quality sleep gives Sukha (pleasure), Pushti (nourishment and growth), Bala (strength and immunity), Vṛṣhatā (potency and sexual vigour), Gñāna (wisdom) and Jīvita (longevity). There will be an increase in the sense of well-being by the rejuvenation of the body and the mind. Sleep will restore the natural equilibrium throughout the body, bringing the three doshas into harmony and balance.

Improper sleep will result in Dukha (grief), Kārśhyam (feeling drained and fatigued), Abalaam (loss of strength and immunity), Klebatā (impotence and sterility) and Agñāna (stupidity and ignorance) and even death. A burning sensation in the eyes, headaches and body aches and irregular bowel movements are some of the ill-effects of not getting enough sleep.

Like a Yogi meditates regularly and consistently to reap the rewards (attaining perfection) of being in the transcendental state, proper and consistent sleeping habits ensure that you will have the gift of longevity, happiness and great health.

The ancient texts have described various types of sleep:
- Sleep from extreme exhaustion or tiredness (this type of sleep can cause Vata imbalances, and all the problems associated with that)
- Sleep because of laziness and lethargy (when you awaken from this sleep you experience brain fog and confusion instead of clarity and freshness)
- Sleep because of illness (may help in recovery, but doesn't really rest the body and mind like natural healthy sleep does)

- Unnatural and unexpected sleep (can signal disturbances all over the body and in the mind, alarmingly, if it continues to be repeated, can portend death)
- Natural sleep which comes at night and is the best and most effective this type of sleep is considered a gift from the Mother Divine. In fact, all the other types of sleep are characterised by Ayurveda as disordered sleep, which need to be rectified.

Additionally, napping (for more than 20-30 minutes) during the day is said to take you towards obesity. Staying awake into the wee hours of the night means that the body doesn't get the time to assimilate the food you may have eaten, leading to nutrient deficiency and all sorts of digestive disorders.

You will find plenty of literature about Ayurveda, and a plethora of books written on the subject, so we will not dwell on this too much. It would be a good idea to figure out your doshas though, and the best way to do this is, of course, to go to a good ayurvedic doctor who knows the art of pulse reading. He/she will be able to tell you exactly what doshas make up your nature, as well as which doshas are imbalanced, and also help you remedy them.

A consultation with an ayurvedic doctor is the best way to remedy recalcitrant doshas. However, here are a few suggestions that have worked well for us and our friends and families over the years. These are by no means comprehensive. Think of them as ayurvedic home remedies.

Handling the 3 Doshas

Whatever your dosha combination, through observation and some practice you will be able to figure out which dosha is disturbed. Any imbalance in your doshas will affect your sense of well-being and the quality of your sleep.

Here are a few generic things you can do to calm down any irritated dosha.
1. Foot massage with or without oil before bed is great for absolutely anyone. The pressure should be such that it is comforting and calming for you.
2. Full body oil massage, even done by yourself to yourself is great. This can be done anytime during the day. Use good quality coconut oil, unless your ayurvedic doctor has asked you to use some other type of oil.
3. Nadi Shodhan Pranyama or alternate nostril breathing —instruction video on **www.booksbybnd.com/sys/media.**
4. A shower with warm or hot water if you are taking the shower towards night is ideal. However, the shower head should be such that it lets out an uninterrupted flow of water and doesn't break it up into droplets.
5. Daily prescribed practice of the Art of Living techniques of meditation—Sudarshan Kriya, Sahaj Samadhi Meditation and Padma Sadhana. Visit **www.inergyworld.com** to know more.
6. Nasya (nasal drops)—Two drops in both nostrils with Anu Taila (medicinal nasal drops) in the evenings can induce good sleep at night. Doing this when you wake up in the morning can reduce the feeling of heaviness and lethargy after improper sleep.
7. Creating feelings of gratitude and satisfaction within yourself just before going to bed is considered by Ayurveda to be greatly beneficial for sleep. Gratitude journaling could be woven into your winding down ritual.

Vata imbalance will mean you will lose sleep easily. The quantity of sleep will not be enough. You may have jerky movements during sleep that could potentially wake you up. You will be a light sleeper.

Vayu Mudra

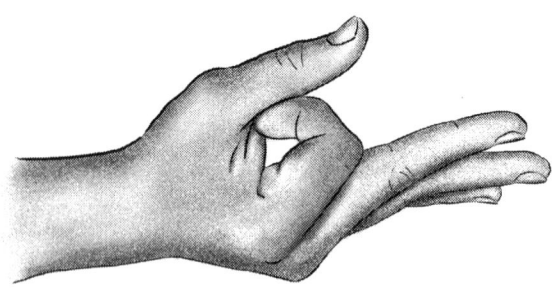

If you feel that your Vata is aggravated, then here are some things you can do to neutralise it.

1. Massage oil on the feet and on the head.
2. If oil is not available, or you don't like oil at night, even a plain head and foot massage is great for calming down Vata exacerbation.
3. Do oil pulling. Half fill your mouth with coconut oil and just hold it in there for 5-15 minutes. Soon your mouth will fill up with a mixture of oil and saliva. Don't give in to the temptation of sloshing the oil around. That will give a different result from what we want. Spit it out and rinse your mouth.
4. You can sit in Vayu Mudra. The first finger curls in to touch the base of the thumb and the thumb rests lightly over it. The other fingers can be stretched out or relaxed, however you feel comfortable. Keep this hand position on both hands and sit. You may do other stuff like watching a movie, listening to

music, talking to people, etc. while you are doing Vayu mudra. It's worth noting that for some sensitive people even watching a movie that has a lot of action and movement can cause Vata imbalance.

5. Stick your tongue firmly to the top of your palette for 2-3 minutes. Then relax for 2-3 minutes. Repeat 3-5 times. This helps calm down a racing mind, among other things.
6. A meal that includes unpolished red rice in the early evening may help.
7. In a country like India, the most natural way to take care of Vata is to awaken half an hour before sunrise. This doesn't mean that you can sleep less than 8 hours. You simply have to get into the habit of sleeping early.

Remember that high speed travel will always aggravate Vata and if you have flown or been in a fast train or car ride, doing even one or two of the seven things suggested above can help a lot in bringing Vata back into balance.

I personally go through bouts of Vata instability and my favourite way to stop this madness from taking over my life is foot massages and the Vayu Mudra.

Varuna Mudra

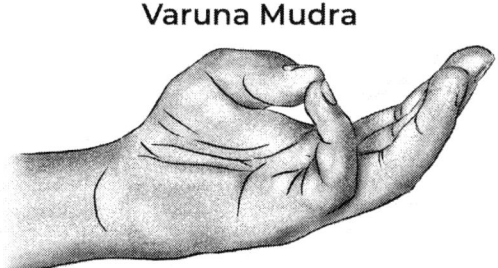

Pitta imbalance creates a loss in quality of sleep. You will not get enough deep sleep. Unstable Pitta can adversely hit the quantity of sleep that you get as well.

To stabilise Pitta, try one or more of these:
1. Vayu Mudra for 5 minutes followed by Varuna Mudra for 5 minutes—the tips of the little finger and thumb touch lightly. The rest of the fingers are stretched or relaxed, whatever makes you feel better.
2. Drink a small glass of warm, organic, reliably sourced, A2 cow milk with a teaspoon or two of A2 ghee in it.
3. Spend time with people you love and with whom you can completely be yourself and relax.
4. Play soothing, relaxing piano or flute music.
5. Play chants like the Devi Kavacham or Hanuman Chalisa.
6. Take a cool shower during the day—warm to hot at night. The shower head should provide uninterrupted flow of water.
7. Cool the bedroom. Use light, pastel cool colours in the bedroom. Keep it muted and elegant.
8. You can play nature sounds—especially sounds of rain, flowing water, sea or waterfall sounds to soothe you.
9. Mild, pleasant fragrances could help as well. Try something like sandalwood, geranium or lavender and see how that feels.

I can get high Pitta episodes, which give me pounding headaches and make me irritable, impatient and angry. The easiest way I know of to deal with this is by simply taking a long, long shower, and following that up with some pranayama and meditation. Sandalwood paste made from real sandalwood (and not some essence or perfume) applied on the forehead helps soothe a headache. Being with people I love brings my pitta crashing down to normal.

Imbalances in Kapha actually cause sleepiness—but at all the wrong times. For normal, healthy people, Ayurveda indicates that while night sleep brings forth the glory of

Prana Mudra

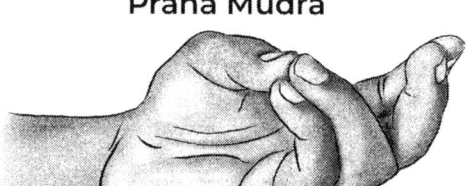

health, excessive daytime sleep can actually initiate a host of unpleasant health conditions. If you feel drowsy during the day, or not fresh when you awaken after a long slumber, an unruly kapha could be at fault.

To fix this, here are a few suggestions:

1. Do moderate to heavy exercise for about an hour between 5 and 7 p.m. This should make you feel pleasantly tired when you get to bed.
2. Eat an early dinner. dinner, definitely 7.30 p.m.
3. Apply a little bit of coconut oil on your body before you take your pre-bedtime shower. During your bath, rub it off. This oil + mild exercise of removing the oil is just perfect to handle the kapha sluggishness.
4. Apart from the Vayu and Varuna Mudras, do the Prana Mudra for 5-10 minutes—the tips of the thumb, little and ring finger touch lightly and other fingers are stretched out or left relaxed, whatever feels more comfortable for you. The Prana Mudra is is a great exercise, especially in the morning, if you find yourself slow-moving and unable to get started with the day.
5. During the day, Bhastrika Pranayama as taught in the Art of Living course, is highly recommended to fight off the urge to sleep at wrong times. Three rounds of 20 reps each are more than enough to wake you up.

6. A dry powder massage of besan (gram flour) + triphala powder in equal proportions all over the body can help shake off the Kapha stupor.

You will find videos with instructions on how to do Prana, Vayu and Varuna mudras, along with some other mudras on **www.booksbybnd.com/sys/media.**

When all the systems of the body are working fluidly, together in harmony, a special type of glow dawns in the body. Your eyes sparkle. You have strength and stamina. There is ample energy. Your mind is sharp, yet relaxed and calm. This is an expression of the subtlest and loftiest forms of the three vital energies—Prana, extracted from Vata, Tejas from Pitta and Ojas from Kapha.

When the three energies are settled and in harmony for a prolonged period of time, then the body catapults into its fullest expression of health and well-being. A soft blush of vibrant bouncy health surrounds you.

The original matrix of the body was created so that it could be in this state. This is how the actual blueprint of the body finds complete expression. And whatever else you do, you cannot achieve this ultimate expression of health in the body and mind without proper sleep.

Good Night!

Babies and Sleep

One of the most frequently asked questions that I encountered while I wrote this book was—I am a new mom. The baby has taken over my life and I don't think I remember what sleep feels like. I am exhausted, cranky and depressed. What can I do? How do I cope with this crazy sleep deprivation? How do I get my baby to sleep?

I normally write about what I have researched and experienced. And I am not a new mom and won't be one, at least in this lifetime. I felt this was a subject that only a mom could talk about with authority. It had to be someone who had been there, done that and dealt with it.

I asked some of the moms I knew and admired, and I present to you their stories—short accounts of how they survived and even enjoyed that precious time when their children were just infants.

Perviz

Many mothers tend to be overprotective of their babies. They don't allow other people to touch them or carry them. Then these kids will want to stick to you 24/7 till they are around 12 years old or so. I don't think you want that, do you?

I had twins, and when my boys came back home from hospital, it was a Thursday. We used to have satsang at home on Thursdays and there were a lot of people in the house. Loud music, singing, clapping, laughing and of course, meditation. Our twins went to each and every person, who held them gently and lovingly, and though the bhajans that evening were extra loud, they slept through the whole thing. I let my babies go to anyone who came home to visit—this helped them become friendly as time passed, and they both developed great social skills, besides giving me an hour or so of rest.

They are 20 now, and I think their social skills are a little too good—too many girlfriends—if you know what I mean. But I digress. Let me get back to when they were just born.

I was lucky enough to have a night nurse during the first month or two. I strongly believe a mother needs her sleep. If you cannot have a night nurse, then someone you trust from your friends' circle or family—your mother or mother-in-law or your best friend—can take over that job at least a few times a week.

You may ask, why not the husband? Well, he had a full-time job and needed his sleep and his energy to function effectively at work. Having said that, I did make my husband take care of the kids on Saturday nights.

I realised that when I had slept well, I could take care of both the boys during the day—and they were quite a handful. Even as toddlers, if things were too quiet in the house, I would immediately know they were up to some new mischief.

My parents and husband, Farida Aunty, Nergish Mami, JD and Zubin, were always at hand to help during those early days—they were my heroes and I will forever be grateful to them. My mother was like an army general. She took charge and made sure everything in the house worked like clockwork. This is important. Have a few people you know you can completely trust around you. There are just too many things to deal with when you have a new baby and being able to unflinchingly ask for help is a blessing. Don't feel shy or awkward. Just ask.

Look after yourself. If you are healthy and strong, you will not collapse and will be able to take care of your baby that much better.

One other big thing to do—when they sleep, you sleep. Don't make the mistake of trying to get other work done while they are sleeping. It will all get done sooner or later. When the baby is sleeping, you too catch as long a nap as you possibly can. What might actually be an hour of peace could feel just like 2 minutes.

Don't take your kids out to movies or rubbish places like that. Take them to a park or a beach. Let them be close to nature as much as possible. Encourage them to play with animals. They turn out healthier. I recently read that when toddlers play about in the mud, they get a lot of good bacteria from there and it develops their microbiome—whatever that is. Basically, they get better, stronger immune systems and don't fall sick so often. And if they do, they recover really fast.

Expect to have post-partum depression. You will feel low and miserable for no reason at all. Breastfeeding helps deal with that. Also, regular meditation and being with the people who love you. This depression thankfully doesn't stay for too long and you will feel like yourself in a few weeks or months. Don't overly concern yourself about it.

Massages helped me a lot. I went and took as many massages as I could. Pamper yourself and keep yourself as happy as you can. It reflects back on the kids.

Breastfeeding is not as easy as it looks. Be kind to yourself. If you are having a problem, then ask for help. If nothing works well for you, then use a breast pump and some sterilised glass bottles. Don't feel bad about it.

Craniosacral Therapy is brilliant for both mom and baby and will help the baby settle into a routine and make breastfeeding much easier if you are having trouble with it.

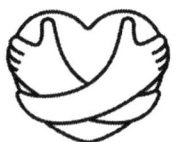

LOOK AFTER YOURSELF. IF YOU ARE FEELING HEALTHY AND STRONG, YOU WILL NOT COLLAPSE AND WILL BE ABLE TO TAKE CARE OF YOUR BABY BETTER.

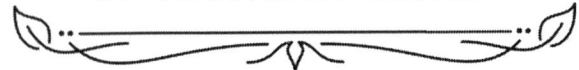

Diapers are God's gift to new moms. Use them, especially at night. Clean the baby as soon as you awaken.

Two things you definitely shouldn't do, at least according to me:

1. Give the baby cough syrup so that they sleep all night, and you can sleep too. There will be nights when you will want to shove a bottle of that stuff down their throats, just so you can rest. Don't do it. Their sleep–wake cycle should be natural—and at least for me and my babies, within 2-3 months, both the boys were sleeping more or less on schedule. I am so glad I didn't give in to the cough syrup temptation and allowed their sleep cycles to form naturally. Of course, if they do develop a cough and your doctor recommends cough syrup, by all means give it—and have a big smile on your face as you anticipate at least a few nights of uninterrupted sleep.

2. Don't get your kids into the bad habit of rocking them to sleep. They will cry, cry, cry if they don't get it and

make your life miserable on a flight or a long-distance train journey.

Lots of people will tell you lots of things that you should or should not be doing. Do not take all the advice. It's so easy to give advice and go. Don't stress yourself out thinking—oh I have to do this, do that … Just relax.

Each of us is unique and different. Our babies are too. See what works for you and your beautiful baby. Do that.

Women have been doing this for millennia. Know that you can, too.

All too soon that cute cuddly little thing will be demanding money to take his girlfriend out to party. And asking all sorts of questions and totally defying you. Driving you up the wall and down the other side.

Enjoy those precious days of new motherhood while you can.

Neha

Most people will sigh nostalgically when you ask them about becoming a new mom. The two things they say are: I was so happy, and I had forgotten what sleep was. It was not so for me. I was happy. And I got great sleep.

Impossible?

Let me tell you how I did it.

When I got pregnant, both my mother and my mother-in-law insisted that my husband and me sleep each night at 10 p.m. Throughout the 9 months of my pregnancy, I had a super strict bedtime. Sometimes I felt I was back in school, the way my mom would rush me to bed as soon as it was 10 in the night.

Amazingly, because we had that habit ingrained within us, when my son Soham was born, the one thing I didn't have to worry too much about was sleep. His sleep cycle, right from the start, synched with mine. I had a night nurse for the first few days and my husband learned from her how to get the baby back to sleep in case he woke up in the middle of the night. He would simply hum a soft lullaby and Soham would soon be fast asleep again. My sleep was mostly undisturbed and great. And because of that, my energy levels were fabulous and I could really take care of my boy.

The other thing my mother used to do diligently was get the baby to pee at regular intervals, even if that meant waking the baby up—seems counterintuitive when you read this—most moms would never awaken a sleeping baby. But doing this meant he hardly ever wet his bed, and the whole nappy-diaper exercise was a walk in the park for us.

Like other moms, I too relied on diapers in the night, and when he infrequently did pee or poop during the night, it was not much of a job cleaning him up when we awoke in the morning.

Because of the super regular sleep times, pee and poop times and feeding times, the first few weeks that seem to be horror stories for other moms were a breeze for me. Literally, the only nights that we were awake were when he was ill.

As I write this, my son is 11 years old now. He goes to bed every night by 9.30 p.m. and wakes up fully rested and rejuvenated the next morning, bubbling with energy for the day ahead. I am pretty sure his great sleep and vibrant energy are directly related to the discipline my mom enforced upon me … and him when he was a baby.

Shefali

I realised how important sleep really was only during my pregnancy, and as a new mother of triplets.

My babies were born extremely premie and they spent the first 10 weeks of their life in the hospital. The hospital would not let us stay the night in the NICU, so we returned home every night. I could not sleep, as I was worried and anxious about the babies and kept dreading that 1 a.m. call from the hospital, saying something had gone wrong. I couldn't take any sleep medication either as I was lactating. I spent the nights of those first ten weeks with a lot of interrupted sleep. I would wake up multiple times during the night, breathing fast and feeling anxious.

But this interrupted sleep was nothing compared to what happened when the babies came home. They were three premie infants with their suck–swallow–breathe reflex still not fully developed. They would take 45 minutes each to take one bottle of breast milk. And, by the time I finished the third, the first one would be hungry again. Also, I lost my father around this time in India, and I couldn't go home. I was in a state of clinical depression, unable to process both my grief as well as my guilt of not being there. Even when I could lie down for a while, I couldn't sleep. I spent multiple nights like that, without a wink of sleep. I was physically exhausted all the time, but unable to sleep.

Most baby books advise new mothers to catch some sleep while the baby is sleeping. I had three babies who rarely slept at the same time, and even though I had a good nanny and a truly understanding husband, I still found it difficult to sleep. This affected my health.

Depression resulted in lack of sleep and lack of sleep worsened the depression. It was a vicious cycle, and I simply couldn't break out of it.

I really don't know how I survived those first few months.

When the kids were four months old, my husband's company had a weekend outing. We left the kids in charge of my mother-in-law and the nanny with great trepidation. We drove from Dallas, where we used to live, to Austin.

We checked into the hotel at around 4 p.m. We had a couple of hours to settle down, and were supposed to meet the gang at 7 p.m. for socialising. This was the first time in four months that we did not have one of the babies in the room. Both Ganesh and I thought we would catch a quick nap for an hour or so. We set our alarm for 7 p.m. and slept. And slept. And slept!

We slept through two alarms, several hotel wake-up calls, calls from Ganesh's colleagues, and woke up straight the next morning at 9 a.m.! It was the most undisturbed, wonderful sleep we had ever had! Our bodies were so sleep-deprived that we could have slept through an earthquake that night.

That one night of sleep did us both a lot of good. We returned to India when the babies were nine months old. It was only then that I could sleep normally. I guess all I really wanted at that time was to come home.

Was there anything you did that helped during that time?

My case was really different. I was a new mom of premature triplets with a very bad case of depression that was a combination of postpartum depression and unresolved grief. I was given anti-depressants, but I chose not to take medication as I was lactating.

I tried long walks, pranayam, yoga—but for almost six months nothing really helped much.

The entire experience did make me realise the supreme importance of sleep, though—something I had never given much heed to, through my life.

I always craved to return to India. It was a deep psychological need for me to 'come home', so to speak. The minute I landed at Mumbai airport, somehow, I already started feeling calmer inside.

Then I went to Goa and grieved for my father. In the US, I couldn't grieve as I had the responsibility of caring for

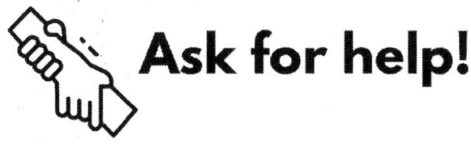
Ask for help!

my three babies. In India, I could hand my babies over to my mother or sister-in-law for sometime, as I grieved and healed. I cried and cried and participated in dad's first annual Shraaddha. That helped assuage most of the guilt.

In India, I had emotional succour—my family, friends as well as hired help. This meant that I could leave the kids for some time with people I trusted. I could work out, go for walks, learn Spanish, write, do all the things I couldn't even imagine doing in the US.

But most importantly, it was the psychological comfort of being 'home', among 'my' people, that helped me sleep better almost instantly. That constant anxiety that used to plague me in the US was suddenly, magically, taken away. Kind of hard to explain. But I could breathe better.

Relief flooded over me as I slowly but surely became myself again—stronger and wiser for the experience. Most importantly, I learned never to take sleep for granted. I consider it a blessing that each night I can sleep well, and wake up rejuvenated, ready to face the challenges of a new day ahead.

My two boys and one girl are strapping opinionated teenagers of 15 and I will soon write a book about how to deal with teenage triplets.

Puja

Oh goodness! Just thinking of those early days and my coping mechanisms makes me shudder. I have a wry smile as I remember what a glorious mess I was when Aarna was born.

Everyone knows just how much I love my sleep. And as fate would have it, my Aarna did not like to sleep. She was what I called a grazer. Just like her mother, she wanted small meals every hour rather than eating, or in her case, drinking 1 or 2 good meals through the night.

Of course, I would have to wake up every now and then to feed her. I simply couldn't bear to see her uncomfortable and crying. The resulting lack of sleep hit me quite hard, and to put it politely, I had many heightened emotions. Kapil, my husband, will tell you all about that, if you ask him. Be careful, though; he can go on and on for a week if you let him start talking about those days …

My mother and my sister Rachana were there with me during that time. They fed me as I fed my baby. You have no idea how much it helped to have them around. They knew what I liked to eat, and made delicious stuff that I gobbled down. Ever so often, they would jump in to take care of Aarna while I caught an hour of peace and rest.

On nights when I couldn't manage, I would wake Kaps (Kapil) up, and after I fed her, Kaps would burp her. He had a particular walk, like a South Korean soldier walking up and down the steps believing that would make Aarna burp and go back to sleep! We had a good burp partnership. Mums know how important it is for babies to burp. Otherwise all the milk comes out and creates a mess—and I don't even want to talk about that.

I had read that being born is a great trauma. You have been floating around relaxed and at peace, everything taken care of for 9 lovely months. Then, you are suddenly and violently pushed out from that haven of tranquillity and have to face monstrous giants who make all sorts of weird sounds at you. Aarna was lucky to have Kaps, who is a brilliant craniosacral therapist, as her dad.

Often, if Aarna was cranky, he would do a hold on our little one, and through his magical touch, she would start smiling

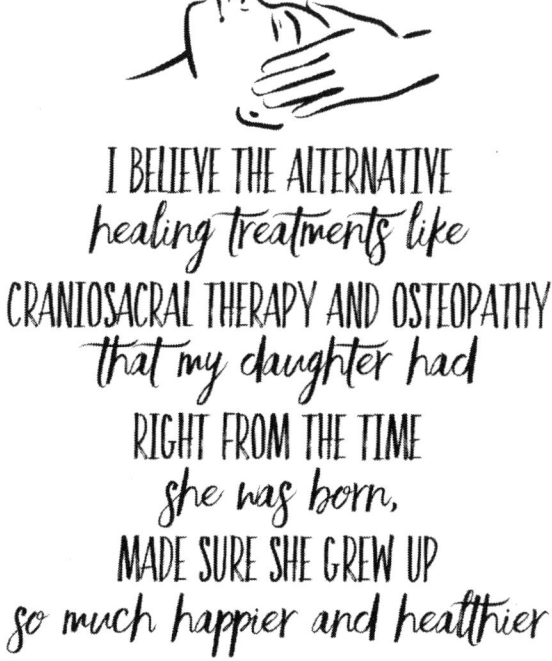

I believe the alternative healing treatments like craniosacral therapy and osteopathy that my daughter had right from the time she was born, made sure she grew up so much happier and healthier

again. Hughette, a great friend and a brilliant osteopath and body worker from Canada, gave Aarna a few treatments while we were at the Art of Living Bangalore ashram. I believe these techniques made sure Aarna grew up so much happier and healthier.

If you can manage it, make sure you and your baby receive these wonderful treatments. You have no idea what amazing long-term benefits these alternative therapies have on our bodies.

Besides the help from Kaps, my mom and Rachana, Sudarshan Kriya and my daily meditation practice kept me more or less sane. Along with this, I made sure I did something for myself every day. Something small that I always loved to do, that would make me feel good. Like watching an episode of *Friends*, or ordering in my favourite food. Maybe getting my nails done or going to meet a friend for a decaffeinated cuppa coffee.

The first 2 weeks I was spending a lot of time in my nightgown or pyjamas all day. I realised that didn't help my mental health at all. This, in turn, didn't help my sleep. I got crankier and crankier. To counter this, I started getting dressed every single day and putting an effort into how I looked. I started taking daily pictures with Aarna, instead of just taking pictures of Aarna by herself, many times posting them on Instagram. That ensured that me and my baby were looking our best.

I realised it made a huge difference to my day if I would even wear a simple tracksuit—just not be in my pyjamas. Then at night, when I changed into pyjamas, it felt more like my usual bedtime ritual to go to sleep. I think this dressing up helped my sleep, and thus my energy levels more than I would care to admit.

It's small things like these that made me feel like I had a more complete day. Then it was not a zombie-like day of going through the motions of feeding and changing diapers because of the sleep deprivation. Oh yes—I made it a point of getting fresh air every single day, even if I was exhausted. Even if it was just a ten-minute walk, I made sure I went out and did it. Being outside gave me a sense of space, which felt great.

It was an exhausting time, but it went fast. It has become a distant jumble of memories, mostly pleasant, as my husband and I watched her grow. My baby is 6 as I write this and she is growing into a beautiful, intelligent, warm and funny young person. I make sure she sleeps on time. Dealing with her long ago taught me never to skimp on sleep.

And me? Thankfully, after the first few months, I was back to sleeping rather well, looking good and feeling great!

Madhushri

Life completely changes when you become a mom. Holding that little angel in your arm for the first time is *the* most memorable moment—you feel you never want to part with the baby, even for a second. You hope that the baby stays the same way and never grows up …

Then reality kicks in. I kept track of feeding and diaper changes and this became an integral part of my daily routine. I made notes of how much milk the baby drank, if the baby was feeding every two hours, how many times did the baby pee and poop, and at what time. I even kept track of how much it pooped—and that was just for starters.

Eventually, you will feel that nothing can gross you out anymore—having been through many smell and sight trials. The wonder of being a mom, the joy of having a baby—all your very own, and the exhaustion and sameness of the routine merge into a blur of days and nights, weeks and months.

This, perhaps, is one of the toughest challenges for a new mom. Even if you have read and researched extensively, the actual experience is something else. I don't think anyone can be prepared for it.

Of course, the first thing that gets impacted is your sleep. You have to wake up every 2 to 3 hours, through the night, to feed your baby. And once jolted awake by the little one's crying, it is incredibly difficult to go back to sleep. At least it was for me. Sleep is an absolute luxury for new moms. I remember not getting 6 straight hours of sleep for the first four years after the birth of my first child! My second was born within just a year and a half of the first.

I recall, just as I would decide to sit and relax, have a quiet meal or take a quick nap was exactly when the baby would decide to start crying uncontrollably. I would have checked that he was sleeping soundly just a minute ago. And of course, somehow only the mom can soothe him. It's like they have a sensor that goes off exactly at the very moment the mom finally manages to put her feet up and relax. I laugh at these incidents when I think back about that time.

IT TAKES A VILLAGE TO RAISE A CHILD

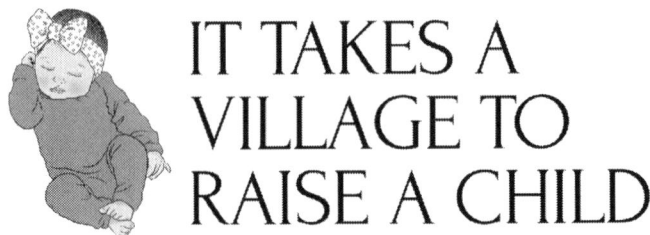

The one thing that helped me the most during this time was my Sudarshan Kriya practice and Sahaj Samadhi meditation. Those 20 to 30 minutes gave me a ton of energy that kept me going through the whole day. I felt so relaxed and calm with the baby (and others too) and I felt it somehow compensated for my lack of sleep.

Finding a quiet space in the midst of all the activity and noise is very essential. The quiet space does not have to be a physical space; it is feeling the silence from within and being with it. This will really help you to embrace and enjoy every moment with your baby.

Time flies so quickly, before you realise it they are all grown up and independent.

I say this to all the new moms—take all the help available to you from friends and family. I was indeed lucky to have amazing support from my husband, mom, mom-in-law and so many other amazing friends who all cheerfully pitched in.

The saying, 'it takes a village to raise a child', is so true.

Mostly, as you are going through the mess you might find yourself in, just know that this time passes very quickly. Cherish it while you can, because, soon, you will have to get ready for bigger adventures with your children.

A few years later, all this will be just a faint memory. And I guarantee that in just a while, you will find yourself telling new moms, 'Don't worry. You will be fine. The baby will be fine. And soon, you will be able to sleep!'

As I write this, my beautiful boys are 8 and 7 years old. They are charming, naughty, funny, exasperating and intelligent all at once, and I wouldn't have it any other way.

Good luck to all new moms!

Prama Bhandari

The trouble with having babies in my time (1960s) was that no one was there to warn you of the actual reality of it. I had no books, videos, etc. to even remotely prepare me for the experience. Neither was there anyone to guide me spiritually or teach me yoga, pranayam and meditation. I had to cope on my own, and I had no idea how to go about it.

I had to deal with lack of sleep and my crankiness as I looked after the baby 24/7. I slept when the baby slept. And my baby didn't like to sleep for long.

There were no Pampers and Huggies, only cloth diapers that had to be washed and hung up to dry on the line. Sheets and mattresses that got wet or dirty had to be washed as well. There was nothing to protect them from the pee or the poop. If you had a son like mine, then there was a daily mound of sheets, diapers, and still more sheets and diapers to be washed and ironed.

So what did I do? I hate to admit this, but whenever I felt overwhelmed (and that was most of the time), I threw tantrums and had quarrels and altercations! And I cried. The only ones to console me were a small golden Labrador pup, who would cuddle up close and lick me, and a gray Persian Angora cat, who took it upon herself to guard the baby, pulling at my sari or nightie whenever he cried.

I have read about husbands pitching in and helping right from the start these days. Not so in the 1960s. One day, when I was complaining about all the diapers filled with potty that I had to wash, Ranji (my husband) laughed and said, 'Well, he's a shitty little thing but he's all our own.' I nearly threw a diaper filled with shit at his face.

I remember immediately sitting down and writing a letter to a friend in America for help. In those days, it took 2 weeks for a letter to be delivered even by airmail. Imagine my joy when a month later I received a note from her, saying, 'Just mailed you 2 plastic panties. Hope that helps.'

So the long and short of it is, I did not cope very well. However, by the time the second and the third child appeared (in rather quick succession), I was wiser, or so I thought. Our youngest always accuses me of helping him like the taste of alcohol, as when I felt overwhelmed, I would take a tot of brandy and then feed him—which made him sleep 6-7 hours at a stretch. But it was not something I could do daily, mainly because I hated the taste of alcohol.

My children have children now, and who knows, I might even become a great grandmother!

Sowmya

Babies cry!

I am a mother of twins and I used to get stressed if my little ones wailed. They kind of did it in turns and left me frustrated and exhausted. I really wanted to do all I could to keep my babies happy. And whatever I did never seemed to be enough. Sleepless nights meant even more tiredness and helplessness. I was a mess.

Until, at one point, I realised that the crying was just part of their language of expression. That's what they do. They coo and gurgle, chuckle and warble, and they cry. It's not such a big deal that they cry. This attitude shift in dealing with a crying baby helped me more than anything else.

As a mother, I did my best to soothe my crying babies. But when I did it without the associated stress it used to create in

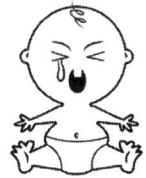

> AT ONE POINT I REALISED THAT THE CRYING WAS JUST PART OF A BABY'S LANGUAGE OF EXPRESSION. THEY COO AND GURGLE, CHUCKLE AND WARBLE, AND, THEY CRY. IT'S NOT SUCH A BIG DEAL THAT THEY CRY. THIS ATTITUDE SHIFT IN DEALING WITH A CRYING BABY HELPED ME MORE THAN ANYTHING ELSE.

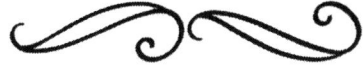

me, somehow things changed. When I dealt with my babies with a sense of calm, I saw that my babies responded.

The more I was cool, unruffled and happy, they were, too. It was an absolute wonder how these tiny human beings could sense my inner peace and effortlessly reflect it.

I am an Art of Living teacher and a Bach Flower therapist now. I can see how meditating for a few minutes and taking a few drops of the Bach Flower remedies could have made life so much easier for me and my babies at that time.

These days, I have helped quite a few moms with the remedies, so they can relax ... and to their delight, as they relax, they see their babies relax as well. When they meditate, their babies settle easier.

And of course, happy, contented babies means great sleep—for the mom and the baby!

With sleep sorted, the rest is usually easy …

Nisheeta

Blue eyes, blond-brown hair and sparkly angelic energy—this was my daughter Elena when she was born. The blue eyes had a sharpness that looked like they could see through you, and a depth that looked like a wise old soul sat behind them. And when those eyes closed, her face could have been of one of the angels in the Sistine Chapel.

She created a stillness as she slept, which spread around the house, enveloping us. Many times, making me slip into sleep as well, along with her.

But to get those eyes to close was one of the biggest challenges I have encountered in life. I remember thinking that this was harder than any career or personal challenge I have ever faced. I had to try different things each time—rock her in various ways, walk around the room holding her (even when my back felt like it was breaking and my knees were about to give way), hum softly to her … and then hope and pray that something would work and she would sleep.

I was convinced that sleep was most important for her, and I hunted for ways to get her to sleep. I discovered Harvey Karp's almost miraculous whispering method (on YouTube—find the link on **www.booksbybnd.com/sys/media**) that worked like magic for Elena. His method comprises of making a unique loud whispering sound while rocking your baby in a certain way.

Interestingly, my European husband was clear that he himself needed to sleep well at night, so that he could function well the next day. He wanted the baby to be in a different bedroom, a distance away, on the other side of our big living room. I wanted the baby to be in our room (as is the case in most Indian families). We converged on putting her in a beautiful bassinet midway—in the living room. If she let out

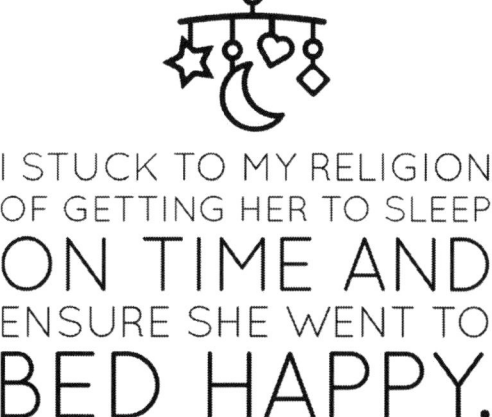

I STUCK TO MY RELIGION OF GETTING HER TO SLEEP ON TIME AND ENSURE SHE WENT TO BED HAPPY.

a soft sound at night, I would immediately awaken and go to her, and his sleep wouldn't be disturbed.

Her sleep was my topmost priority. My own sleep was secondary. But during the times she napped during the day, I either slept or meditated. The Yoga Nidra by Gurudev Sri Sri Ravi Shankar became my lifeline, during her naptimes, giving me deep rest and healing my own body over many months post delivery.

The days and nights rolled into each other, and I think the only personal priority for me during those early months was doing the Sudarshan Kriya and Sahaj Samadhi meditation every single day.

My commitment to a 'sleep calendar' helped greatly. I diarised her wake time and sleep time. Every nap and every time she slept was recorded. I could see a natural rhythm emerge. All I had to do was find a way to get her to sleep/nap on time, and she would awaken on time, bubbling with energy.

As she grew, I stuck to my religion of getting her to sleep on time and ensure she went to bed happy. As she invented new delay tactics, I kept inventing new steering-to-sleep tactics that challenged my creativity to the hilt.

She is the nicest natured child. Sleep for her and meditation for me have worked better than I dared imagine. She has been happy, vibrant, endlessly fun and content. She is my wish fulfilled.

Anuradhika

New mum?

Do this!

Make sure you have support

You are going to be depressed. There, I said it.

You will have moments (and days) where everything looks grey and miserable.

Despite the joy of seeing our newborn, there were times when I would burst into tears for no reason. It had nothing to do with my baby, and everything to do with my hormones.

Luckily for me, my husband, my mother and my grandmother all understood. They supported me, comforted me, and I was able to give my body the time it needed to heal. Please make sure when those tears come that you have someone, anyone, who will hug you and love you and tell you it's all going to be okay.

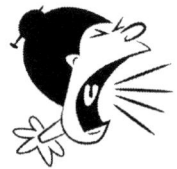

SLAP ANYONE WHO TELLS YOU MUMS SHOULD BE HAPPY, MUMS DON'T CRY, MUMS ARE NEVER UPSET. BECAUSE LET ME TELL YOU, THEY MAY NOT ALWAYS BE HAPPY, THEY DO CRY A LOT AND SOMETIMES THE SMALLEST OF THINGS CAN UPSET THEM.

And slap anyone who tells you mums should be happy, mums don't cry, mums are never upset. Because let me tell you, they do.

Get some sleep and take care of yourself first
I know this is going to raise eyebrows, but if you don't take care of yourself, you won't be able to take care of your baby. Sleep when your baby sleeps. That to-do list can wait. You need sleep—end of story. Make time for yourself, fit some me-time into your schedule. Trust me, no baby has ever suffered because mum took some time for herself!

You will make mistakes—and your child will still live and grow up to be fabulous
Why does everyone, including the mom herself, expect the new mom to be perfect? I know I read every book there was to read (those from my generation will definitely recognise Dr Spock, Penelope Leach, and *What to Expect When You're Expecting*), and got advice from every aunt (and uncle) under the sun. But when my baby was born, I was so exhausted and overwhelmed that I could barely remember my name, forget all the pearls of wisdom I'd read.

And so, of course, no matter what I did, or how I did it, there was a better way of doing it.

And so, the comparisons start.

Did I know that so and so was such a perfect mom? Clearly I was not up to the mark!?

Did I know that such and such had a baby who NEVER cried—unlike mine, who screamed blue murder at the drop of a hat?

My advice? Drop 'perfect' from your vocabulary and ignore all the comparisons and advice. Accept that you will make mistakes, but you'll still be an amazing mother—trust me.

There is only one you, and you are perfect as you are.

Ask for help

You are perfect the way you are, but you're going to be exhausted mentally and physically. Asking for help does not mean you're an incompetent mother. It just means you acknowledge your limits.

I was so lucky to have my mum and grandmother there for me for both babies.

Have someone around whom you love and can trust to look after the little one while you take some time off to rest.

All the best!

Shavina

I had my baby when all my friends' children were teenagers.

I was fortunate that Aadya was a baby that loved her sleep. She would effortlessly slip into dreamland and stay there through the night, without a single whimper or a howl. I used to feed her at around 11 p.m.—just before going to sleep myself—and I think that did the trick. At 6 a.m. a tiny yelp would awaken me for her next feed.

I have a little technique that I simply must share with all moms.

Babies often wake up crying in the middle of the night because of colic. I have a 'desi nuska' (traditional Indian home remedy) to handle this. As soon as any signs of discomfort or irritability are seen, apply a pinch or two of hing (asafoetida) heated in a teaspoon or so of desi ghee to the baby's belly button. A little dab of this great stuff on the baby's toe nails seems to help in getting the baby back to cooing and smiling.

Don't ask me how it works. I am a mother, not an ayurvedic doctor.

It is not a Farex baby, but a well-rested baby who is a happy and healthy baby. And well-rested babies mean well-rested moms.

Good Night!

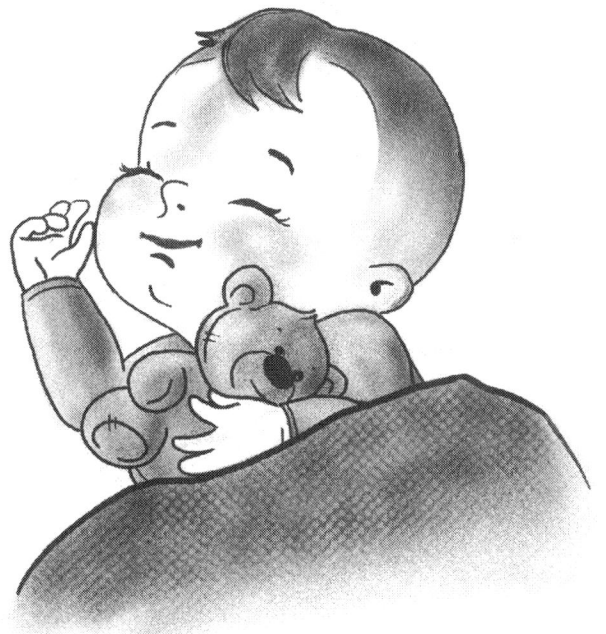

Miss Mystery

Last heard, Sherlock Holmes hadn't found the key,
Neither had Poirot cracked her age-old mystery.
While finding things, Nancy Drew sure lost a bit of it,
Maybe Tintin caught some, tackling the 'blistering barnacles' bit.
I wonder whether Einstein pondered on her or not,
Since she gives a ton of 'energy' and does 'matter' a lot.
Relatively speaking, time and space don't seem quite right,
When you are travelling with her at the speed of night.

Did Newton never get hit on his head with her hammer?
Was his bed's gravity strong enough to attract her glamour?
Did Pythagoras know that to have success fair and square,
It needed the 'triplets' of smart work, deep sleep and a prayer?

Did Archimedes have a eureka moment, soaking in her embrace,
Or did he simply threw in the towel, to abandon her hypnotic chase?
Did Heisenberg have uncertainty about his relationship with her,
Or for him, was her position or her momentum always a blur?!
Did Sigmund, when different layers of our conscious mind strip,

Study how sleep affects them all… or did she give him the 'Freudian slip'?!
Was she included in physiological needs in his 'hierarchy' by Maslow?,
Or was she studied in 'classical conditioning' by the dog loving Pavlov?!

There have been great men and women in recorded history,
Who championed sleep, unravelling her sophistry,
And others with their disruptive genius inventions,
Inadvertently spoiled our nighty restful dimensions.

Did Gutenberg in 1450 know, when he invented the printing press,
Allowed wisdom to travel, but good books put sleep time in regress?!
Will Graham Bell realise, with his invention of the telephone,
Connect lovers across seven seas, yet did sleep dethrone?!

Did Edison or his son know, that designing of the electric light,
Powered countless social changes, but vandalised the night?!
Did the creators of the airplane, television or computer ever know,
They'll interlink our world, make it small, but produce sleep woe?!

We are grateful,
To them all, for the greatest developments seen by humanity,
Yet, we need a degree of discretion to sustain our sanity—
Our ability to timely switch off 'lights, camera and action',
So that we can safeguard 'success and sleep satisfaction'.

—Dinesh Ghodke

Frequently Asked Questions About Sleep

1. **How do I set my bedtime? How do I figure out what is the best time for me to go to bed?**
   The best way according to me is to take a 15-20 day vacation into nature—some remote place where there is no internet and dodgy electricity at best. In a few days of being there, with nothing much to do towards evening, you will begin to feel sleepy at your natural genetic bedtime. Some people will want to turn in by 8 or 9 p.m. Others by 11 p.m. or so. Yet others will stay up till 2 a.m., counting the stars. You can consider this to be your perfect bedtime.

   The challenge is not so much in finding out your ideal bedtime as it is in maintaining it once you get back home. This little vacation will do all the other systems of your body a world of good as well—as you begin to function more in synchronisation with the natural rhythms of the earth.

2. **I am a shift worker. What can I do to fix my sleep?**
   Quit the job. This is the best solution. Do it now.

   If you are in emergency services and quitting is not an option, then the next best thing to do is to ensure you have bright white lights in the place you are working in—maybe even get a sun lamp. Ensure you give your SCN artificial signals that it is still daytime. As soon as you finish working, wear dark glasses and go back home to a bedroom that is darkened with blackout curtains.

Give yourself some time to wind down before hitting the bed and weave as many points from the 'Winding Down Ritual' that you can into your routine. Essentially, you need to fool your brain into thinking that night is day and day is night. Maintain this even on the weekends.

3. **I fly through different time zones many times a year. My sleep is disturbed. What should I do?**
   For each time zone you cross, your body requires one day to recalibrate itself. If you have done a long-haul flight over several time zones, then plan to stay for a longer time in that place. Second, start to follow the routine of your destination 3-4 days before you fly. Third, when you land, right away follow the routine of the place you are in.

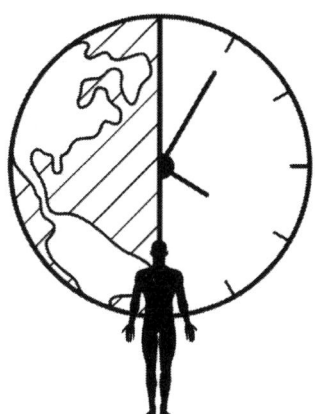

YOUR BODY CLOCKS RESYNCHRONISE THEMSELVES TO ADJUST TO A NEW TIME ZONE AT THE RATE OF 1 OR 2 TIME ZONES PER DAY

During the flight, stay hydrated and drink a LOT of water. Avoid alcohol or anything with caffeine in it. Maintain the sleep–wake routine of the local time at your destination during the flight.

Yoga, pranayama, meditation and Sudarshan Kriya (especially the long Sudarshan Kriya that is done under supervision of a qualified Art of Living teacher), once you land, will help to adjust to a new time zone quickly. Seek out an Art of Living teacher or a centre from **www.artofliving.org**.

If you know how to trace your meridians, then trace your meridians 3 to 5 times based on your current time zone as soon as you land. This can help minimise the effects of jet lag. If you wish to learn more about the meridians and how to do meridian tracing, check out **https://bawandinesh.in/alternative-healing/**.

If you are a pilot or an airhostess, then do all the things listed in question 3 in addition to following all the tips set out through this book. Be zealously consistent and regular with your yoga and meditation practices. A shielded, blacked out room to sleep in is non-negotiable.

4. **I drink alcohol or take a sleeping pill to sleep. Is that okay? If it's not, what should I do?**

   Even if you manage to fall 'asleep' after having alcohol or a sleeping pill, the sleep you experience is not true sleep. You will not reap the benefits of natural, restful sleep if you rely on any sort of alcohol or pill. You are getting forcefully knocked out—quite different from sleep. In consultation with your doctor, and only as the doctor advises, wean yourself off any sleep medication you may be on. There are some excellent sleep doctors who can help fix sleep disorders—seek them out and take their help.

Follow the tips and techniques in this book and it will not be too difficult, especially if your sleep issue is because of poor lifestyle choices.

Find a good homeopath, ayurvedic or siddha doctor to aid you. Alternative healing methods like Craniosacral Therapy and the Bach Flower Remedies can benefit you in ways you cannot imagine—not just for better sleep, but for creating an overall sense of well-being. You can find craniosacral therapists trained by Dinesh, me and Dr Ankita Dhelia on our website, **www.sstcha.com**.

You can read more about the Bach Flower Remedies from **www.bachflowers.in**. I teach the Bach Centre UK certified courses. To learn about these almost magical remedies, I would sincerely invite you to do a workshop with me.

Alcohol, in general, is a bad idea. Get off alcohol and choose to get into life positive practices like yoga, meditation and exercise. By the way, if you are one of those people who say—I am not addicted to alcohol, I can give it up any time, then do so right away. If you cannot, it means you are indeed addicted. If you require it, seek professional help to kick this habit. Everything in your body will thank you.

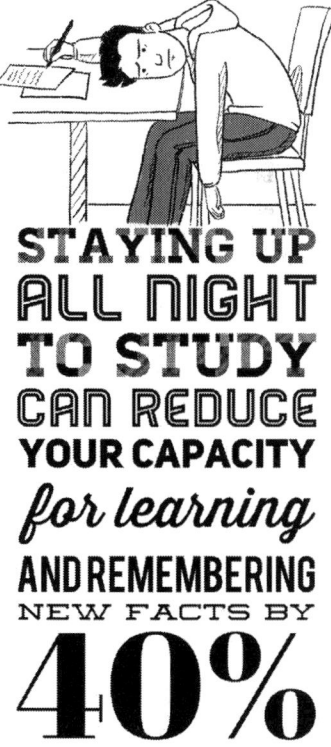

STAYING UP ALL NIGHT TO STUDY CAN REDUCE YOUR CAPACITY *for learning* **AND REMEMBERING NEW FACTS BY 40%**

5. **I feel sleep is a waste of time. I could get so much more accomplished if I didn't have to sleep. And I know that I can get by on less than 8 hours of sleep. 6 hours is more than enough for me. What would you say to this?**

   When you are drunk, you know you are drunk. However, when you are sleep-deprived, you don't know you are sleep deprived. You cannot figure this out at all. To compensate for your lack of sleep, your body will take micro naps throughout the day. You will find yourself drifting off to la la land. In a meeting or an interview, this could be funny at best, or embarrassing at worst. If you are driving, a three-second sleep interlude could prove disastrous.

   Get this in your head. Whatever it is that you are accomplishing in your waking hours, you are able to do it because you slept. If you get 8 to 9 hours of good quality sleep, you will become far more efficient, creative and productive. You will be less moody and grumpy. Like I have said many times in this book, you will feel younger, look sexier, become healthier and be smarter.

   If there is just one thing you take away from this book, let it be this: Sleep is NOT a waste of time. You can indeed *Sleep Your Way to Success!*

6. **I wake up in the middle of the night and cannot go back to sleep easily. What should I do?**

   If you are waking up to pee, then drink water more than an hour before bedtime. Just before sleeping, I sometimes feel dryness in my throat. I just take a few sips of water and that's enough. Just before going to bed, it may be a great idea to go pee.

   If you woke up because of something else—a bad dream, or some noise, or the power went off ... and cannot fall asleep, then the first thing to do is get out of bed. Don't spend time in bed tossing and turning. The one thing we don't want is your mind associating your bed with anything other than rest, sleep and feeling wonderful. While sleep eludes you, you can choose to do whatever you want to—read a book, answer emails, clean the fridge, play some game ... until you start to feel sleepy again. Then get back into bed and go to sleep.

Dr Ankita Dhelia has a fantastic way to deal with this—she always keeps a list of things that need to be done, but are boring and tedious to do. If she awakens in the middle of the night and cannot go back to sleep, she just starts one of those dull, uninteresting tasks that need to be completed.

One of the two things happen—the work is so dreary that she starts feeling sleepy and in a few minutes heads back to bed. Or if sleep doesn't favour her, then at least that work that she had been postponing for ages gets done!

A win-win situation!

7. **I wake up around 3 a.m. feeling completely fresh. After that, I potter around and do some work. Soon I feel sleepy again and go back to sleep for a few hours more. Is this okay?**

Yes. This is perfectly okay. It's a throwback to our time when we were chiefly into agriculture. We would routinely wake up very early in the morning, then do the chores that needed to be done at that time. We would then go back to sleep and wake up a little later, once the sun was up, and resume our day.

My own grandparents used to do this every single day. My granny would be up by 4 a.m. or so and there would be a clanging of pots and pans in the kitchen as she would cook the meals for the entire family for the day. Once she was done, she would promptly go back to bed and be fast asleep until almost 8 a.m. Meanwhile, my grandpa, who was a philatelist, would carefully air his stamps and work on his stamp albums in that quiet time just before dawn. There would be no one to disturb him while he did this delicate work. He would go back to sleep around 6 a.m. and wake up at 8.30 to get ready and go to work.

This phenomenon is called having two sleeps and is quite common and natural. Don't try to change it. Just figure out what you will do when you wake up so early. I would use that time for some thinking and actioning the big goals of my life. It's a beautiful, silent time, perfectly suited for deep thought and decisive action.

8. **I wake up at the slightest sound. Is there anything I can do to sleep better?**
Waking up because of sounds in your environment is quite natural. Through the millennia, sounds in the environment spelt danger and the brain developed this survival mechanism to protect you from getting killed, eaten or robbed.

Waking up because of the slightest sounds simply means that your nervous system is highly strung. Your brain is registering danger and waking you up to deal with it.

Calm yourself down by doing some pranayama, yoga and meditation. The simplest way to calm yourself is to breathe deeply 15-20 times, always ensuring you exhale longer than you inhale. Throat gargles and humming are simple ways to activate your vagus nerve—the one that's responsible for relaxing your nervous system and soothing it.

Slowly chanting mantras like Om Namah Shivaya or Om Namo Narayana will help you relax and unwind as well. Over time, chanting will make your nervous system robust and not easily alarmed, and you will be able to sleep through a thunderstorm.

9. **Once in a while, I need to get up early in the morning for a flight. It's not possible to wake up naturally at that time. I will have to use an alarm clock. Is there some efficient, safe way of rousing myself from deep sleep using an alarm?**

There are going to be times when you need to be up earlier than your usual wake up time. You may have a flight to catch, an interview to prepare for, or any other urgent task. If that's the case, here is a little hack for you.

Remember that the progression towards deeper states of sleep is from awake to N1 to N2 and from N2 to either N3/4 or REM. Similarly, when you awaken, you need to transition to full wakefulness only from N2. When you wake up from N2 sleep, you will usually feel amazingly refreshed and energetic. On the other hand, being yanked awake from N3 or REM sleep can be disturbing, and will leave you feeling tired, disoriented and groggy until you go back to sleep again. Remember, too, that one sleep cycle is approximately 90 minutes.

Say you need to get up at 6 a.m. and you're planning to sleep at 11 p.m. It takes most people between 15-30 minutes to slip into slumber. Your first cycle would start at around 11.30 p.m. Let's divide your sleep into 90-minute chunks.

11.30 p.m. to 1 a.m.
1 a.m. to 2.30 a.m.
2.30 a.m. to 4 a.m.
4 a.m. to 5.30 a.m.
5.30 a.m. to 7 a.m.

Looking at this, it's not a good idea to wake up at 6 a.m. You are going to be in the middle of a sleep cycle, and waking up at this time will make you feel terrible throughout the day. In this case, it will be much better to wake up half an hour earlier than you planned—at 5.30 a.m. Amazingly, with half an hour less sleep, you will be far more alert and refreshed than if you forced yourself awake at 6.

A bit of math like this for certain days when your schedule is a little disrupted will ensure a fantastic day ahead.

Certain scientists disagree with this. Their advice is to clock as much sleep as possible. However, I have personally experimented with this, on myself and many others, and found it to be remarkably effective. Try it out for yourself and see if it works for you.

Always remember that this is a hack and should be used once in a while, and only when waking up naturally is simply not an option.

10. **I like napping in the afternoon. If I nap for an hour or two in the afternoon and sleep less at night, is it okay?**
Unfortunately, the answer to that is a no. I too love my afternoon naps, but sleep science says it's best to limit afternoon naps to between 15 minutes to a maximum of half an hour. If you go over half an hour, then you will wake up from the nap feeling groggy, instead of rested. Besides, a longer nap will interfere with your natural sleep at night.

Ayurveda has an interesting take on naps. Here is a list of people who are allowed naps in the afternoons according to ayurvedic texts:

Those who sing a lot (can't figure out the why for this one!)

Those who study excessively

Those who indulge in too much sex

Those who routinely do heavy physical work

Those who have travelled long distances

Women in their monthly menstrual cycle

And, of course, those who are ill, or are recovering from illness, or who are struck with grief or fear, or feeling melancholy.

Conclusion: If you want longer afternoon naps, take up opera!

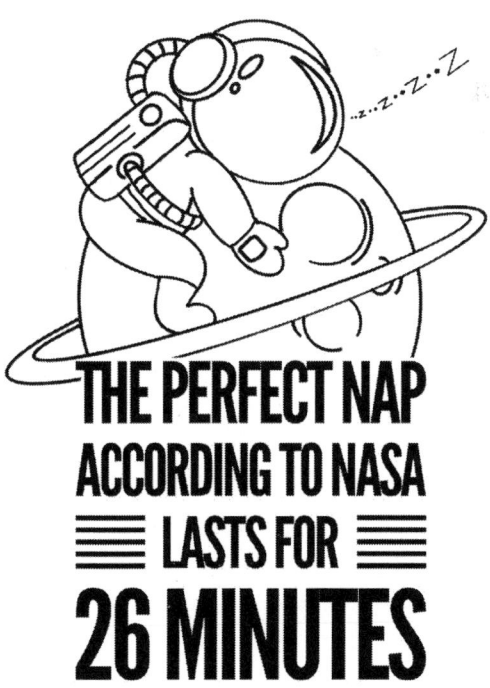

11. My husband and I both work full day jobs. Once our kids are in bed, and before going to sleep, our winding down and relaxation consists of watching some nice TV serials or a movie. It's our time together. You say, we shouldn't have white light exposure at night from a TV or other screens, especially before sleep. What do we do?
P.S.: These days, the TV serials feel more interesting and relaxing than sex. So, please don't tell us to have sex ☺

It is quite unfortunate that watching TV is considered by the two of you as your 'time together'—it's not! It's your precious time squandered on your TV. You say it is relaxing. I would say it is mind-numbing at best—and an unnecessary agitator at worst. The white-blue light from the TV will play havoc with your SCN, delaying your natural sleep cycle. You will feel sleepy much later than you ideally should. Your delayed sleep will mean your early night rejuvenating sleep will be compromised.

This translates to waking up with aches and pains, and not feeling rested, even if you managed to get 8 hours of sleep, which you mostly will not. I can almost guarantee that you will sleep just 6-7 hours—if you are lucky. This means that you are ageing faster than you should—perhaps that's why you feel that TV is more interesting than sex.

I get it that you are tired. But once you have got the kids into bed, this is your time together. Make the most of it. You could plan a family vacation. Sit and talk about your dreams. Think about how you will spend time once you retire. Think of the big life goals that you have, and what you can do to realise them. Chalk out some action plans for the next day, week or month.

Cuddle up and rekindle that earlier romance.

Yes, doing that may feel like an effort at the moment. But it's an effort worth making. Gurudev Sri Sri Ravi Shankar once said that a mature relationship is like an old shoe—comfortable and secure, but with hardly any sparkles. A new love is all bubbly and bright, but has no security. I would say that with a bit of work, an old relationship that is comfortable and secure can be made to sparkle as well. That old flame is waiting to be kindled back into a fire.

And it can all begin with selling off that TV!

12. **I normally get into bed at 2 a.m. and wake up at 10 or 11 a.m. I don't feel rested even though I slept my prescribed 8 hours. I feel I should sleep earlier, but if I get into bed at 11 p.m. like everybody says I should, then I toss and turn and cannot get sleep, and end up even more frustrated and tired. What can I do to set an earlier bedtime for myself?**

If you are habituated to sleeping at 2 a.m. and one fine day you get into bed at 11 p.m., you are inviting frustration.

You need to take this slowly. Get into bed 15 minutes earlier than usual. For you, this will be 1.45 a.m. Sleep may or may not come. Keep doing this for a few days until you sleep off within 10-15 minutes of hitting the bed. It normally takes a week to 10 days for the body to register a 15-minute adjustment.

Now, move your bedtime up by another 15 minutes—to 1.30 a.m.—like earlier, sleep may or may not come. Keep to this new time until it's easy for you to sleep within 10-15 minutes of getting into bed.

Over a few months, continue this process of moving up your bedtime by around 15 minutes and giving your body a few days to adjust to this new sleep time until you get to your desired bedtime.

13. **How to get into bed and fall asleep within 5 minutes?**
   Sleep science says if you fall asleep in 5 minutes or less, there is something wrong!

   You are either overworked or you don't get good quality sleep. If this happens once in a while, there is nothing to be bothered about. If you habitually crash within minutes of getting into bed, some lifestyle changes might be required. Read our book *Happiness Express* for more tips on creating a sense of well-being within yourself.

   You should ideally take between 5-20 minutes to fall asleep. That being said, each person is unique, and if you are waking up naturally without an alarm, feeling refreshed and rejuvenated when you awaken in the morning, and this feeling lasts till noon, please continue doing whatever you are doing. It's suiting you!

14. **How to sleep when you have pain in the body?**
   If you follow a sensible lifestyle (read our book *Happiness Express* to know what I mean)—eat green and healthy, exercise, meditate and sleep enough, the chances of developing chronic pain are minimised. Life, however, does happen, and you may injure yourself or suffer from a painful health condition. If the pain is unbearable, seek professional medical advice on how to handle it.

   I remember when I had popped a disc in my lower back, I was in excruciating pain. At that time, I would lie down as comfortably as I could, and then begin to meditate, and through meditation, slip off into sleep.

See if any of the traditional remedies work. Balm, hot compresses, oil massage—all can help.

Earthing will greatly alleviate pain—check the chapter 'Art of Waking Up' to learn more about earthing yourself.

Another interesting way is to acknowledge that pain, and not try to wish it away.

Focus attention inside yourself, to the area of pain, and become completely aware of it—figure out words to describe it—think of what shape it is, or what colour it feels like. Is it big or small? Is it smooth or rough? Pain is the body's cry for attention, and when proper, deliberate attention is given, you will see that it subsides.

You may say these four short sentences, with all the sincerity you can muster to that part of the body that is troubling you—I love you. I am sorry. Please forgive me. Thank you. Sounds weird, but don't dismiss this technique until you try it.

Osteopathic and Craniosacral Therapy techniques can help tremendously. So can the Bach Flower Remedies if the pain has an emotional root to it.

From your heart, pray to a higher power to relieve you of the pain. You will be pleasantly surprised at how effective prayer can be.

15. **Dreams are inevitable. What can I do to ensure I have pleasant dreams and not nightmares?**
There are quite a few things you can do:
a. Eat a light dinner at least 3 hours before you sleep. Heavy, difficult to digest, extra spicy or sugary food can give you bad dreams.
b. Don't watch or read about anything unpleasant or disturbing about 2 hours before you sleep. Give your mind a chance to wind down.

c. Wear loose comfortable clothes. Sleep in a warm cozy bed in a nice cold room.
d. Sleep in an east–west direction. Many people who complain of horrifying dreams sleep peacefully and calmly simply by changing the direction of their beds.
e. Sometimes the place you are sleeping in can give you

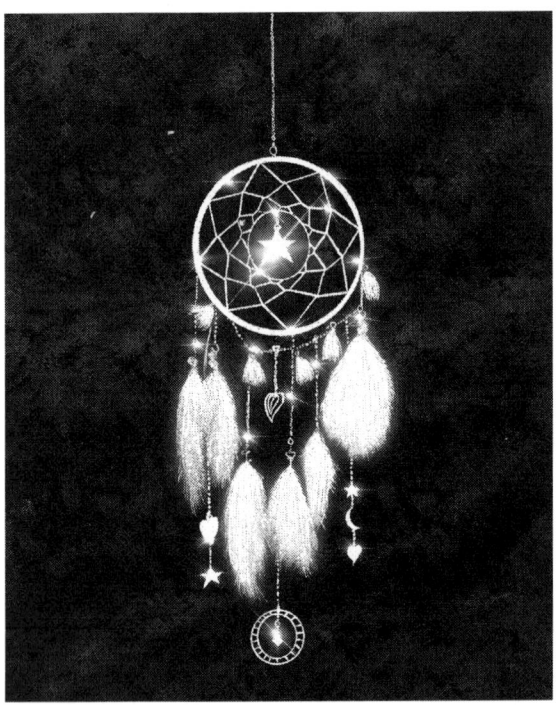

unpleasant dreams. Especially if something violent has happened there. I remember being in a beautiful hotel room and not getting good sleep and being plagued by vague violent dreams. After two days, I got my room changed and could immediately sleep really well.

I found out later that someone had been raped in the previous room. If you suspect something violent has happened in a new house you have moved into, a few Vedic Poojas can set everything right.

Check the website **https://vaidicpujas.org/** for more information about the different poojas or homas that can be performed to create positive vibes in your home.

16. **Mosquitoes are enemies of good sleep. Any natural solutions for them?**

Mosquitoes are enemies. Period.

Did you know that more than a million people die every year because of mosquito-borne diseases? Mosquitoes are a bane for humanity and should be eliminated.

My experience is that they tend to get inside your room towards evening. Around 4 or 5 p.m., tightly shut all the doors and windows of your bedroom. Reopen them in the night if required. Keep low lighting in the bedroom—mosquitoes are attracted to well-lit rooms.

It's not a good idea to use sprays with chemicals to kill them or those mosquito mats that may contain harmful substances in them. It is far better to try out traditional ways of finishing them off.

1. **Camphor:** Close all doors and windows and light camphor—the strong smell of camphor drives mosquitoes away. Within an hour or so, there won't be any mosquitoes to bother you. I like to hang little packets of camphor around my room. If you like the smell of camphor, this is a brilliant little hack.
2. **Garlic:** Boil some garlic for a few minutes and let it cool. Put the liquid in a spray bottle and spray your room. Garlic can get rid of mosquitoes. Maybe that's why mythology says that garlic repels vampires.

3. **Lavender, mint and tea tree oil:** All these three beautiful fragrances are anathema to mosquitoes. Use dabs of essential oil around your bed to keep these pests away. A combination of lavender, mint and tea tree oil in a spray bottle filled with water squirted in and around your room also works.
4. **Basil leaves:** Basil leaves kill mosquito larvae. Plant some basil at the entrance of your home and in your garden. Mosquitoes and their pestilent offspring will die. Besides, you will have a fantastic organic source of basil leaves for your pesto, soups, pasta, salads and pizzas.
5. **Neem leaves:** Burning neem leaves gets rid of mosquitoes. I personally cannot stand the smell of this and it gives me a headache. But the mosquitoes are gone.

17. **Are there any optimal sleep positions?**

Yes. There are.

We have all experienced a few aches and pains when we wake up after sleeping awkwardly. I recently learned at a workshop that if we sleep awkwardly or in an incorrect position, certain parts of the body get blood-deprived, while others get too much blood. This could lead to major imbalances over time, wreaking havoc on our system.

People sleep in a variety of ways, but there are only three optimal positions.

The first: Lie flat on your back, legs a little apart. Hands can be by your side, palms facing up, or on your stomach or chest. Your shoulders should be on your pillow such that your head is on the pillow and your neck is well-supported. Around 1.5 inches of your shoulders on the pillow would ensure this. Most people, including me, would use the pillow only to rest the head and leave the neck without support. Try this one, though. It's so comfortable that you'd wonder why you didn't do it all your life!

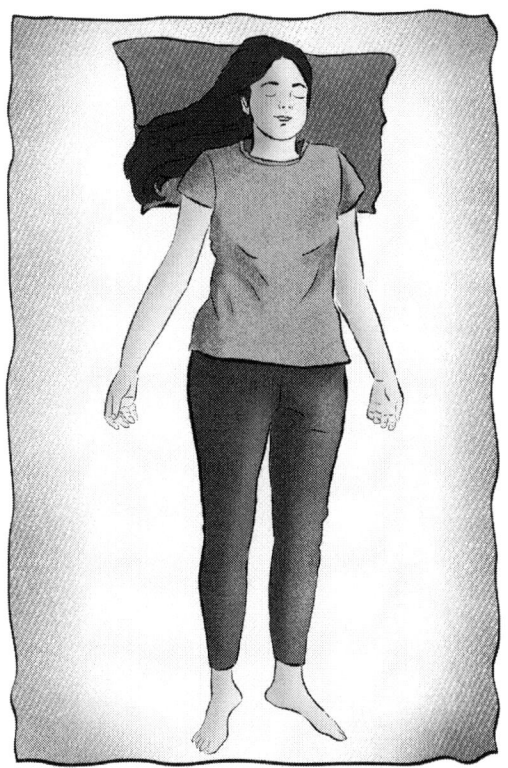

The second: Turn to your right side. Your head should be on the pillow, but your shoulder shouldn't. Your left hand should rest on top of the left side of your body, reaching somewhere near your hip. Your right hand should be bent at the elbow, palm upwards near your face. Your legs should be bent comfortably at the knees so that the heels of both legs are in line with the base of the spine. You may have another pillow between your legs if you wish.

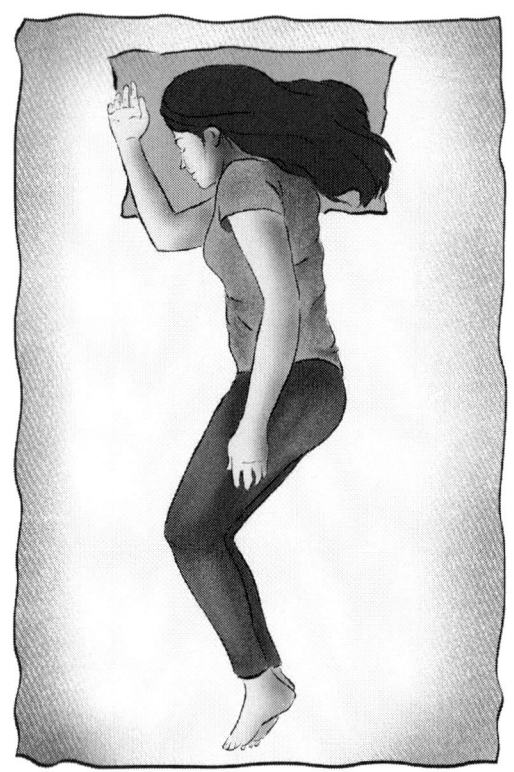

The third: Mirror image of the second, with you turned to your left side.

Do not sleep with your head towards the north or south. Instead, let your head be in the east or west. Though there isn't much scientific evidence supporting this, and many claim that it doesn't really matter, I have found that lying in the east–west or west–east direction helps me sleep better and experience nicer dreams. Moreover, there are many references in our scriptures that say keeping the head towards the east is the best position.

You are probably wondering how one can manage to sleep through the night in only those three positions described above.

The answer is simple: by deciding to do it. There was a time when I would sleep with three pillows. One under my head, another over it and a third one between my legs. After a workshop on sleeping better, I resolved to change this habit. The effects of a lifetime of incorrect sleeping positions vanished within a few weeks.

The body is far more intelligent than you can imagine, and when you start doing what's good for it, you will be astounded at how wonderfully cooperative it can become.

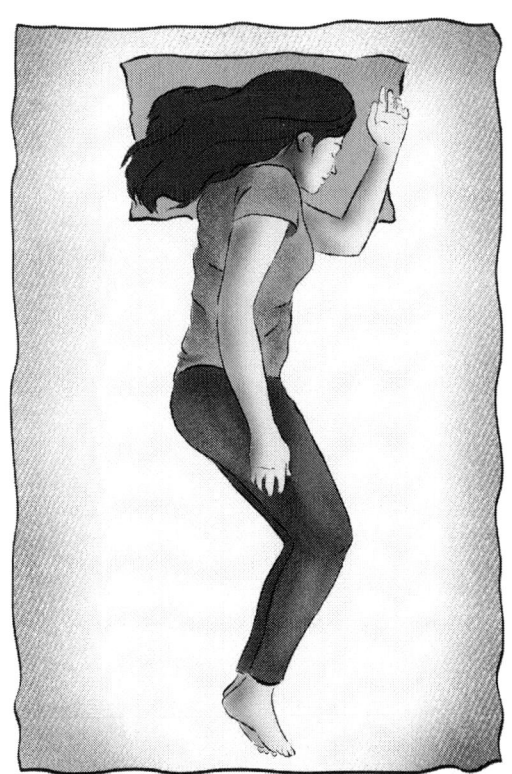

18. **I snore. Quite loudly, I am told. So loudly that sometimes I actually wake up because of the noise of my own snoring. What do I do?**

There are quite a few natural remedies that can help you stop snoring. Don't ignore loud snoring. This type of snoring can be a precursor to other far more serious sleep and health disorders like sleep apnea, insomnia or obesity. These conditions bring with them a host of related issues that can make things really unpleasant for you. Try out the remedies listed below and see which of them work for you.

If nothing works, consult an expert sleep doctor who may be able to help you sort out your problem.

Lose weight: People who are overweight are twice as likely to snore than those who aren't. The extra fat around their necks narrows their airways, causing them to snore. The easiest solution to eliminate snoring is to lose a couple of kilos. Clean up your diet by cutting down on inflammatory foods, clock in some exercise and ensure you are giving yourself at least an eight-hour sleep opportunity each night. Hopefully, not only will the snoring stop, but you will feel healthier and fitter.

Change sleep positions: Lying more on the back while sleeping can cause more snoring. Have an intention before sleeping that you will turn towards your sides as you sleep. This little intention is usually more than enough. Read about the sleep positions outlined above as the answer to the seventeenth question.

Stay hydrated: Drink more water during the day. Dehydration will cause mucous formation in your nose which will make you snore. Six tall glasses of water each day would do you a world of good. As a side note, it is worth noting that if you are feeling thirsty, you have already been dehydrated for a while

Tape your mouth shut at night: I know—it sounds weird. Don't discount this simple technique until you try it out. You may need to experiment with different types of tapes until you find the one that you are comfortable with. Google 'sleep tape' for ideas. Various people talk about various ways of taping the mouth at night—figure out the way that's most comfortable for you. The first few nights it may bother you and you will want to remove it after a few minutes. It's okay to do that. In a while, you will get used to it. I have friends for whom absolutely nothing worked and they did taping and have managed to dramatically cut down their snoring.

Practice nasal taping: Stick a tape around halfway on the bridge of your nose (check how to video on **www.booksbybnd.com/sys/media**) can help a lot as well. I know a few people who do only nasal taping and not mouth taping and say they manage to sleep through the entire night and awaken feeling really fresh.

Breathing through your mouth instead of your nose can cause many unpleasant health conditions, of which snoring is just the tip of the iceberg. Taping not only helps you snore considerably less, but will contribute to your overall health and well-being as you are forced to breathe through your nose.

Chewing: Chew your food. Each morsel you put in your mouth needs to be thoroughly pulverised by your teeth—and that takes 30–50 chews. Eat food with more fibre so you are forced to chew. A big percentage of the digestion of what you eat happens in the mouth. Chewing helps assimilate the nutrition from your food and as you chew your way to health, you will strengthen your jaw muscles. These muscles help keep your mouth shut as you sleep. You will breathe more through your nose, which means you will snore less or not at all.

It's quite amazing to know that chewing your food well can help you and those around you sleep better!

Singing: When you sing, you strengthen your tongue and the throat muscles. With stronger tongue and throat muscles, the chances of snoring are dramatically reduced. Treat yourself to a solo concert in your shower or when you are driving. If you don't sing too well, be considerate and do it while you are alone.

Take steam: Inhaling steam with a drop or two of eucalyptus or tea tree oil in it can clear up a stuffy nose and handle many allergens that could be causing you to snore. Heat water to its boiling point and, carefully pour it into a big vessel. Sit comfortably and bend over the vessel such that your face is above the steaming hot water. Cover your head with a towel. Take long deep breaths in and out for as long as you can—at least for 2-5 minutes.

Quit smoking and alcohol: Drinking alcohol, especially before bed, relaxes your throat muscles and causes you to snore. Smoking causes inflammation in your throat tissues and makes you snore. Besides, both these habits will only cause you more and more problems as time passes. Quit. Right away.

If you have a partner who snores and their snoring is disturbing your sleep, then an extreme solution is to sleep in two different rooms.

19. Are melatonin patches safe?

Melatonin triggers the sleep cycle, prepping your body to unwind and gradually drift into slumber. Melatonin also prevents you from feeling gloomy and blue. Our body has a vast and supremely sophisticated chemical system that regulates the production of melatonin and all other hormones. The body creates all these chemicals in the perfect proportions that are required from moment to moment. No external agency can match this perfection and is likely to create some sort of problem.

For whatever reason, if your body is not producing enough melatonin, then your ability to sleep and enjoy the benefits of sleep will be compromised. The best way to fix this is through as natural a way as possible. Try the Bach Flower Remedies, Craniosacral Therapy, Ayurveda, Homeopathy or other alternative healing methods.

If you still require a temporary boost to your melatonin levels, just so things can normalise in the body, then a melatonin patch may help. As soon as you feel that your sleep is returning to a sort of normalcy, discontinue the use of the melatonin patch. Don't get habituated to using it over prolonged periods of time.

It is our personal belief that it is never a good idea to get that it can make naturally into the habit of putting anything into the body on a regular basis. If you continue to pump the body with stuff that it can intrinsically make, from outside, the body learns a bad habit. It feels it doesn't need to make that substance anymore, and may even shut down production completely, creating an unhealthy dependency.

20. Are there sleep-related benefits of bedtime stories for adults?

As your body prepares to sleep, the mind needs to wind down and relax. If there are too many thoughts jumping around in your head, then it becomes that much more difficult to fall asleep.

A well-written bedtime story distracts the mind and gets it involved in its universe and plot. A pleasant short story with a satisfying end can calm and soothe you after a full day of work.

When you choose to read something at bedtime, make sure it doesn't agitate you in any way. That would defeat the purpose. The last thoughts you have at night are more or less the first thoughts you awaken with. Be careful what thoughts you sleep with—they will be running around in your head for eight or more hours.

A comforting, quieting story can relax jangled nerves, and ease an agitated mind. It can make you smile, bring on feelings of hope and gently nudge you away from your own worries and concerns.

You will definitely sleep better.

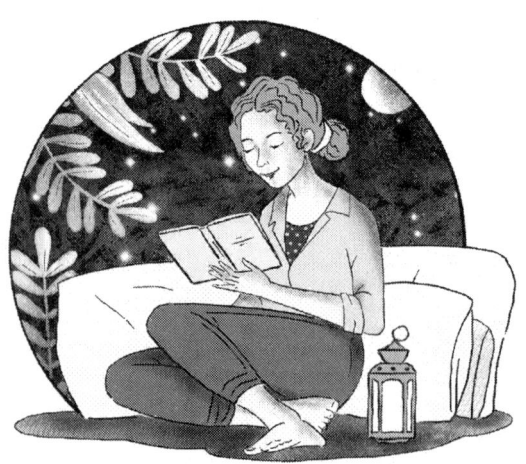

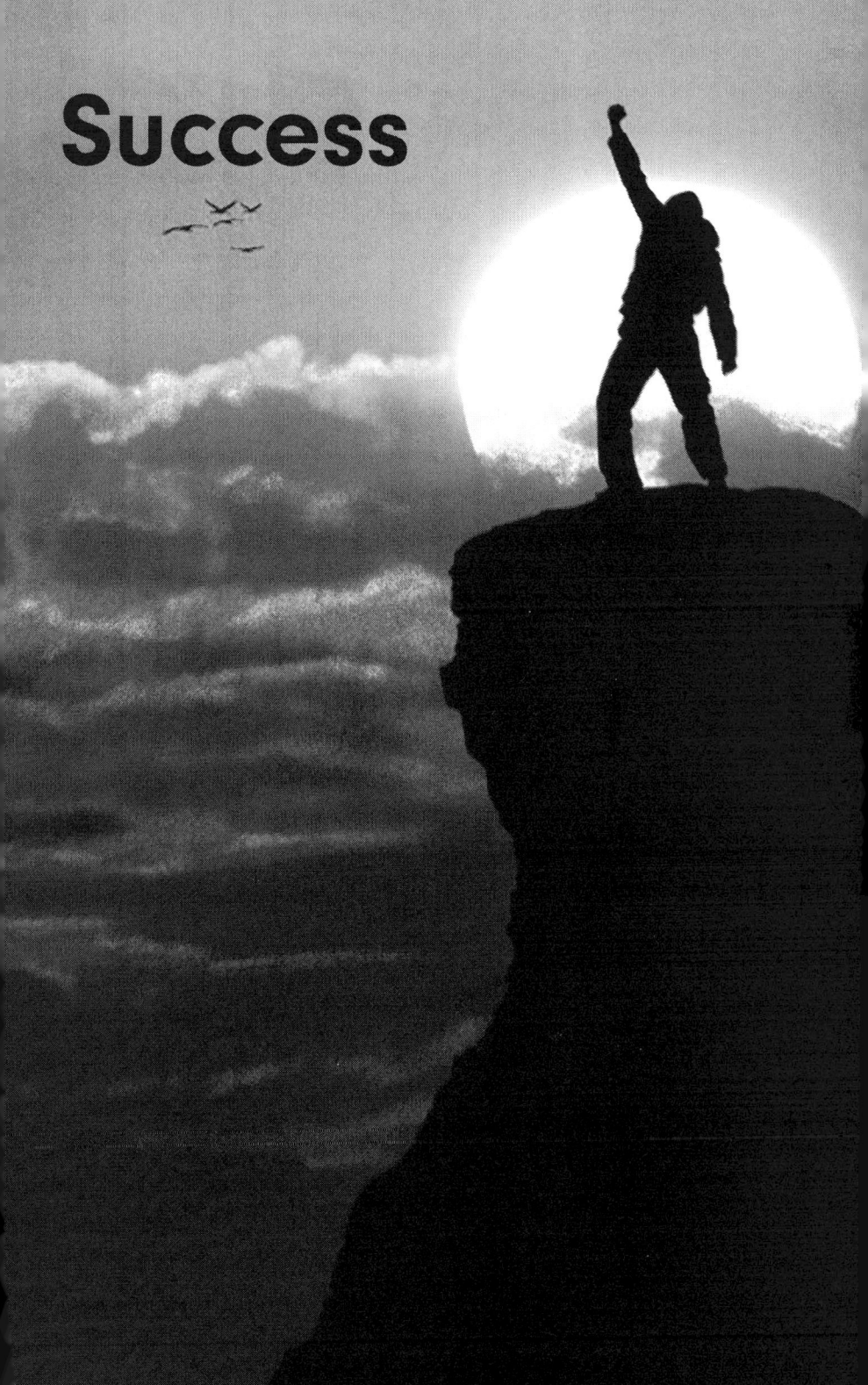

The Monster in Your Head

It had been a long day. Multiple protracted Zoom sessions in which I had to talk a lot meant that by evening, I had a sore, burned-out throat. Every night, our friend Sunny who was staying with us would come up to my room and massage some oil on the soles of my feet for a few minutes—this reduces Vata and allows one to sleep better.

That night after he had finished, and before I went to bed, I felt I needed to do something for my throat, as I had a marathon session of Zoom calls the next day as well. My favourite go-to remedy for anything throat-related is taking a few drops of propolis tincture. It stings, but the next day the throat feels healed. Propolis is a resinous, waxy substance made by bees, and when tincturised, considered to be really good for the throat as well as for other itches and wounds.

Sunny asked me what I was having, and I asked him to open his mouth and popped in a few drops. He made satisfactory groaning and moaning noises as the propolis burned its way down his throat. I laughed and got into bed.

The next day, bright and early, he came to my room and exclaimed that it was the best night of sleep he had had for a long time—and asked what the name of that sleep medicine I had given him the night before was.

Sleep medicine?

Those drops that burned me, that sleep medicine, is a miracle, he bubbled.

He said that he was a light sleeper and almost anything that went bump in the night woke him up, but the previous night he had slept peacefully and deeply.

I told him that the 'medicine' was for the throat and had nothing to do with sleep.

He looked confused. 'How come I had great sleep then?' he wondered.

He had firmly believed that this was some magic sleep medicine. His mind had made him believe so, and he had slept well.

Fooling the Mind

Our minds are incredibly powerful and play a huge part in shaping our reality. It is not unusual that if someone believes something strongly, they will be able to manifest it in their lives.

It is quite easy to fool the mind and create what is called the 'placebo effect'. This effect has been featured in thousands of studies and, in fact, when a new drug is released in the market, its efficacy is tested against a placebo. More than one-third of the people in a control group will respond to a placebo, which could be a small sugar pill. People report to have dramatically reduced levels of pain, they stop vomiting, their diarrhoea disappears, long-term migraines vanish, they sleep better and even manage to cure themselves of incurable diseases with a teeny bit of sugar. All because they truly believe that the 'medication' they were given can cure them of their ailments.

This effect can have disastrous consequences as well—people have died from non-poisonous snake bites for example, because they believed that the snake that bit them was poisonous, even when the marks on their skin clearly show the teeth marks of a non-poisonous snake. Yet the swelling and colour of the skin there, as well as the symptoms they die of, are that of a poisonous snake. They die because they believe they have been poisoned.

My grandfather died of a sudden heart attack. Only they found later that it was not a heart attack at all. It was just gas. He felt a lot of pain in his chest area, thought he was having a heart attack and died. His belief that it was a severe cardiac problem killed him. Unfortunately, he didn't know that because the stomach and heart are neighbours, when something is amiss in the stomach, the heart can act up. Some simple home remedy to fix the gas could have cured him in a few minutes … tragically, his belief and his mind killed him.

Monster

If what you firmly believe in actually manifests at least one-third of the time in your life, maybe it would be a great idea to give some consideration to the thoughts that are going around in your head.

What kind of thoughts do you have? What are your beliefs?

Do you think you are not good enough? That you don't deserve what you have got? That you are humdrum and mediocre? That you will never be rich? That everyone else is better than you? That you are prone to failure?

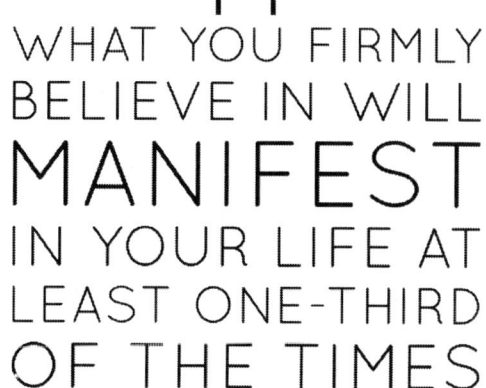

WHAT YOU FIRMLY BELIEVE IN WILL MANIFEST IN YOUR LIFE AT LEAST ONE-THIRD OF THE TIMES

That you are unlucky? That you fall sick often? That no one will ever love you? That you will never get that promotion? That you cannot be happy? That you simply cannot sleep well—whatever you do? That success is something that happens to others ... not to you?

The monster in your head will tell you all this and more. It will say stuff like—*There is no point. You are never going to get what you want. Might as well give up and forget about it.*

It will tell you to cheat on your diet. *Go on. Eat that cake. Anyway, you will never have a healthy, fit body. Might as well enjoy life.*

It will make you skip your exercise. *The whole body is aching. It's so tiring. I hate sweat. You will never look sexy.*

It will make you spend more than you intended to. *Come on. Buy that ridiculously expensive watch. Doesn't matter that you have five more like it at home. You can always take out another loan.*

It will make up all sorts of really good excuses why you simply don't have the time to meditate. Or study. Or work. *I am tired. I am bored. I don't feel like it. Even if I meditate, I get angry. I study so hard and still get terrible grades. I work and work and others are promoted. Not me.*

It has a habit of stretching the negative and disregarding the positive. If you go to a new city and are 'taken for a ride' by a local rickshaw driver, it tells you to conclude that all the rickshaw drivers in this city are crooks. It makes you overgeneralise and magnify unpleasantness. When you experience something pleasant, it will convince you that this was a one-off, a coincidence.

When something goes wrong, it is *always* like this.

When something works out, it's a fluke.

We could go on, but I am sure by now you have a wry smile on your face as you are reading this.

If these are the kind of thoughts you regularly have, and as we saw earlier, there is a high probability that at least a third of them will materialise, is it any wonder that things are the way they are in your life?!

Here is the good news, though. Just as the mind is capable of manifesting the obnoxious, it is perfectly capable of manifesting what you truly desire as well. You do need to train that monster, and make it work for you, instead of against you.

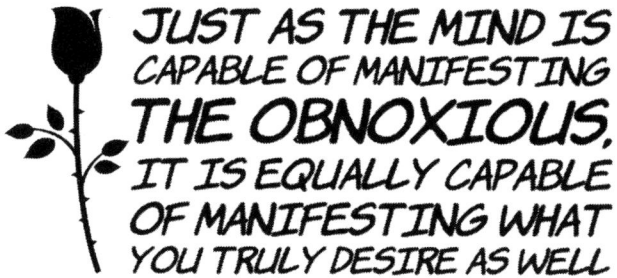

JUST AS THE MIND IS CAPABLE OF MANIFESTING THE OBNOXIOUS, IT IS EQUALLY CAPABLE OF MANIFESTING WHAT YOU TRULY DESIRE AS WELL

When you first begin to deal with the monster, you will find that effortless awareness generated by true spirituality helps tremendously. You will notice that if you meditate regularly, you will catch yourself just as you begin to indulge in that sabotaging self-talk. And already 80% of the battle is won.

Think of the monster as a spoilt child. With a little bit of discipline, it will learn to behave. You cannot wish the monster away. It is your monster. Your baby. Acknowledge it, and then learn to deal with it and train it.

For example, if it says, *eat that cake*, say to it, *yes, I will. Just not now. Later*. That throws it off, and it will not bother you about the cake for sometime.

If it says, *don't bother exercising*, say to it, *just for today, I am going to do it*. It will sulk, but it will agree.

Use this technique to talk back to it. Say *not now, later*, for anything that it tempts you with. Don't make the mistake of telling it a no. It doesn't accept a no. But it will be fine with *yes, we will do it later.*

If it tries to stop you from doing something you know you should, simply say to it, *let's just do it today. Tomorrow we will see ...*

You do this enough times, and you will see that it will soon stop its unrelenting opposition to what is positive. If it tried to overgeneralise the negative, say really? I don't think so. Challenge it. Laugh at it.

As you do this, and stick to doing what is life enhancing—guess what—your life slowly but surely starts to improve ... and the monster in your head will have less and less stuff to complain about.

Its loud incessant stream of negativity will turn into a trickle of whispers. Confidence, appreciation, peace, love, faith, friendship, laughter, hope, beauty, health—all those things you have always wanted will begin to dawn in your life.

How I Handle My Anger

Even though I have meditated nearly every day for almost three decades, anger does visit me once in a while. It's not about not getting angry. The game is all about not staying angry. A stone thrown in a still lake will cause ripples. The point is how fast the ripples die down, not about the ripples being caused in the first place.

When I am irritated or angry, I notice how my monster starts its tirade. I smile at it, and then wish the absolute best for whoever bothered me. I wish they attain enlightenment. If they get

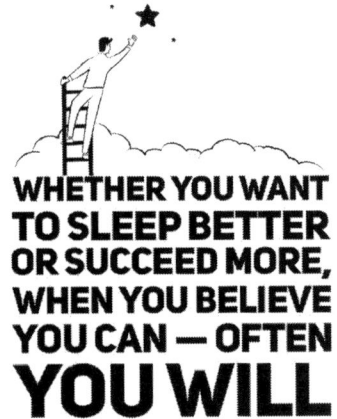

enlightened, then they will definitely stop bothering me—in this life as well as all the others to come! Instead of wallowing in sorrow, resentment and bitterness, and thinking how I can get back at them, I send great wishes their way … and get on with my life.

Whether you want to sleep better or succeed more, when you believe you can, most often you will. As this life supportive circle of belief and manifestation becomes stronger and stronger, failure and setbacks will bother you lesser and lesser.

The monster in your head will be your friend. The incredible power of the mind will be yours to play with. Have fun!

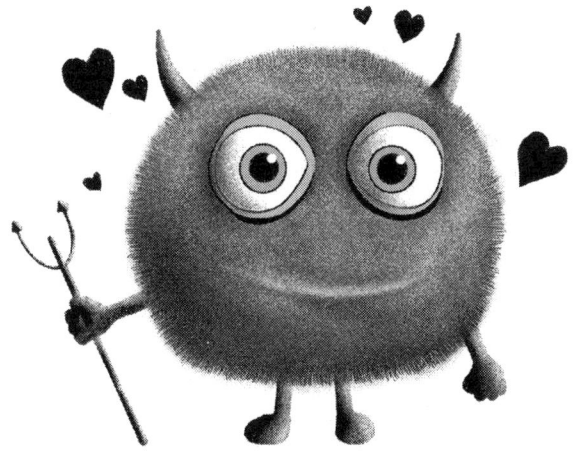

The Pizza of Life

It can be really difficult to get to where you want to be when you have no idea where you are going.

This is a do-chapter. Not a read-chapter. Settle yourself down, get two or three large sheets of blank paper and three pens of different colours, put aside a few hours and only then start reading this chapter. If this is not possible at the moment, just skim through it and come back to it later when you do have the time.

On your paper, draw a BIG circle. And divide it into 8 parts.

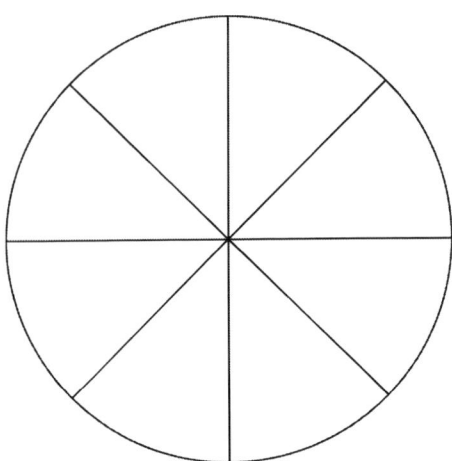

In each sector, write a significant area of your life. Finances, Career, Spirituality, Hobbies, Family, Social Relationships, etc. are some examples. Think about this for a bit. For some people, relationships could be two or even three categories—relationship with wife, relationship with children, relationships with other close friends and family, for instance.

You may have more than 8 categories—that's okay. Just list them next to the circle. If you end up with a lesser number than 8, break up a category to make the number at least 8. A circle with all 8 categories and some spillover could look something like this:

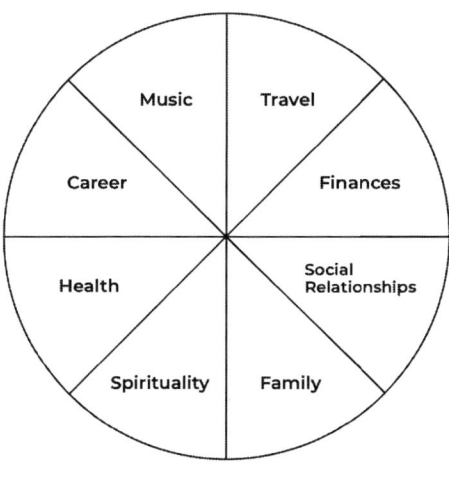

Learning New Things - 9
Helping Others - 6

Next, rank each of these areas of your life from 1 to 10, where 1 means you are disgusted with yourself, you are at absolute rock bottom, and 10 means you consider yourself truly remarkable in that area—it's practically perfect.

These numbers represent your perception of how you feel about yourself in each area. Draw arcs at appropriate places in each sector to reflect your ranking. When you are done, your circle is going to look something like this. It would be a good idea to use a coloured pen to write the numbers and draw the lines.

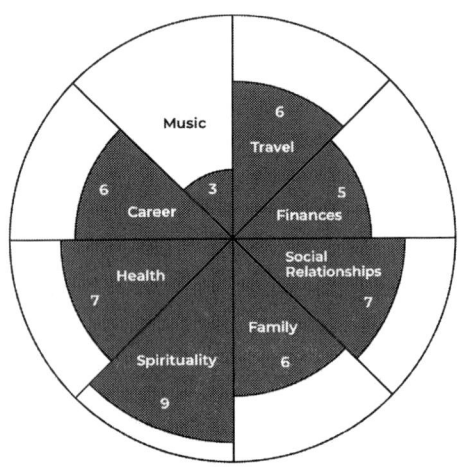

Learning New Things - 9
Helping Others - 6

The next step is crucial. Force-rank the sectors in the order you feel their importance in your life. If you feel, for example, that health is the most important, then give it rank 1. If family comes next, give family rank 2, and so on.

If two sectors feel equally important, you have to choose one over the other. Just for ranking purposes, think about it this way—if you have one, you cannot have the other; then which one would you choose? Rank the one you chose higher than the other. Continue until you have ranked all the sectors. Use a different coloured pen to put in the ranks, so it is clear to you what your satisfaction levels are and how important a particular area of your life is to you.

If necessary, redraw the circle so that the first 8 ranks are in it. The rest can be listed next to it. This step is not really required but fulfils my need for neatness and clarity. ☺

In the illustration, the numbers inside the sectors represent satisfaction levels and the bold numbers outside represent priority.

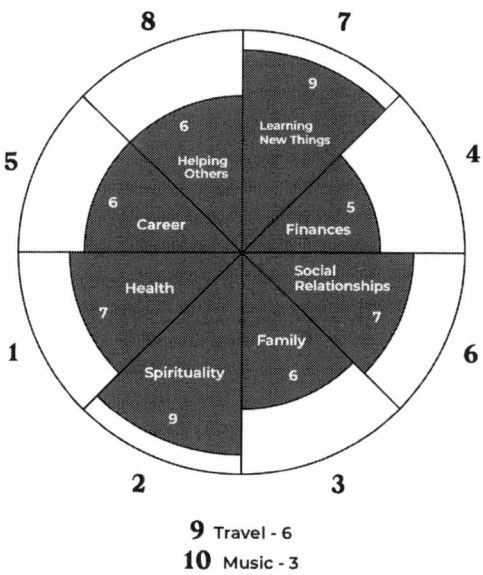

9 Travel - 6
10 Music - 3

Bring your attention to rank 1—check your rating there. There are two possibilities now:

Your rating is 8, 9 or 10.

If this is the case, fantastic! You only need to maintain this score.

Your rating is less than 8.

Take your time and think of how your life would be if your rating there was an 8 or above. Write out what you would be doing, how you would look, what you would feel, where you would be and who would be with you ... Fill in as many details as possible. But don't just sit and think about it. Write. Write. Write. Write the essay out in the present tense, like it has already happened. Coaching research shows that when you do this, it dramatically improves your probability of actually creating that reality.

Now repeat the process for whatever is on your rank 2. Do this for the first three or maximum four ranks where your rating was less than 8.

In the example above, I would do it for Health, Family, Finances and Career. My Spirituality rating is anyways at a 9, so I only need to ensure I maintain it.

By the time you complete this process, you will have 3 or 4 essays written in the present tense about how your life would be if you could manage to get your ratings to an 8 or above in the three or four most important areas of your life according to you.

Read those essays a few times. Mindmap them if you would like to. Add in details if required.

Achieving Versus Being

If someone offers you a fish curry and you refuse, saying you are trying out a vegetarian lifestyle, this would be quite different from you saying, 'I am a vegetarian. I don't eat fish.' The first is superficial, the second is who you are. Contemplate this in this context of your essays. I hope you have realised by now that this is not about achieving some goals. It's about becoming that type of a person. It's not about learning to cook. It's about becoming a chef. It's not about losing weight, exercising and eating right. It's about being healthy.

In light of your essays, give deep thought to these questions: Is this kind of a life worth having? Do I truly want to become this person?

Until the answer to these questions is a resounding YES!, keep at the process. You might feel you want to change your priorities while you mull over this. That's perfectly fine. Make whatever changes you need to and do what it takes to get to that YES! as an answer to those questions.

It may take longer than an hour or two. It could take an entire weekend. Or two. Or three. Stick with it and complete it to your satisfaction ... knowing it is always going to be a work in progress.

When you have finished, you will have accomplished what very few have done. Figured out where you want to get to in life, and who you want to be. Also, how it will be when you get there and become that. And whether you really want to get there and be that in the first place.

The Regret Loop

At this point, some people I have coached get stuck.

They begin to what-if.

They fear that after putting in all the planning and struggle and hard work towards achieving what they wanted, what if they get there and figure out this was not what they wanted in the first place.

What if they regret those decisions they took a few years ago?

This what-iffing stops them from getting into action.

They become victims of analysis paralysis. They plan. Then they plan again. Then they what-if. And plan yet again. They keep on with these mental gymnastics and grow old.

Dreams remain dreams.

In the present, as you create your Pizza of Life, trust that you have taken decisions in the best possible way that you can. Given your life circumstances and the data available to you, what you have decided to create for yourself is your best plan.

And until that future has been created, there is no way you have of knowing whether it is something you want or not.

Think about it this way. You go to a fancy restaurant and check the menu. When you decided to go there, you already knew it's going to dent your wallet. Everything looks delicious and everything is exorbitantly priced. Considering that you couldn't possibly eat everything on the menu and you do want to enjoy the experience, you take your time to order your dinner.

There may be a few things you could do here to make the best possible choice—call up someone you know who has been there before—and ask them what to order. Google the restaurant, check out reviews and see what others have enjoyed most. Ask your waiter for suggestions—possibly even call in the chef—and have a chat with him.

At some point, after all this, you will order your meal. And hopefully enjoy it. Or not.

If you did enjoy the meal and felt it was worth every penny, great.

If you didn't enjoy the meal and regret your choices—thinking you could have ordered something else, or maybe even gone somewhere else—this is in retrospect. There is no way you could have figured this out as you entered the restaurant. You ordered the food with the intention of enjoying the meal, with all the data you had at that point. If the food was not good, then you know if you ever come back here again, you will try something else—or not visit that restaurant again, and try someplace else. These decisions can be taken after ordering and tasting the food—not before.

If you dilly-dally on taking action with regards to your Pizza of Life, it's like going to the restaurant and not ordering food at all because you fear that the food might not be good and you will waste your time and money. It is only when you actually taste the food that you can figure out if it was worth it or not. To taste the food, you have to order. You have to take that risk. Not ordering is not an option really.

At best, you will love the experience. At worst, at least you will not be hungry.

I tell my clients that it is far better to do all that is required to get out there and achieve a dream than sit and regret about what could have been. The sooner they get into action, the sooner they will know.

If it turned out to be what they wanted, fantastic!

If it didn't, at least now they really know and can move to something else. And just for the record, whether they wanted

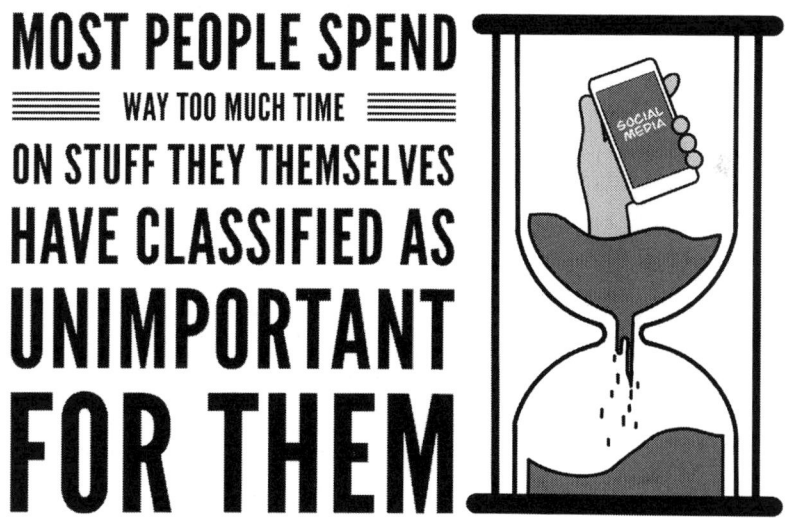

what they got or not, the journey towards accomplishment is a phenomenal teacher. When you know how to create reality from one dream, you will have learned the technology of creating reality from *any* dream. That, in itself, is worth everything.

Action

To dramatically improve the quality of your life, all you now need to do is figure out how to improve the Pizza of Life scores. This translates into creating a step-by-baby-step action plan that will help you get to where you want to be, and who you want to become. And finally, get down to the nitty-gritty of actually executing your plan with small actions consistently, every single day—until one day you wake up to the life you have been dreaming of, and become that person you had decided you wanted to be.

What about the other sectors?

Once you have managed to raise the scores of the three most important ones to you, repeat the process for the next three. Meanwhile, continue to do whatever you are doing so you can maintain the scores on all the other sectors. As time goes by, certain other priorities could pop up, replacing ones you had originally put in. That's fine. Keep moving, adding and deleting whatever modifications to your plan that are required.

When I run this process with clients I coach, most of them are astounded when they begin to see and comprehend the power of their Pizza of Life. The one big realisation they get is that they have been spending way too much time on stuff that they themselves have classified as unimportant and hardly any time on what they feel really matters to them in their lives. It's quite an a-ha! moment. It is in this moment that they begin to realise the actual possibility of creating the reality they have only dreamt of.

Then it's just a question of coherent planning, unswerving execution and easy agility in case life's circumstances force you into a modified version of what you wanted.

And enough good quality sleep.

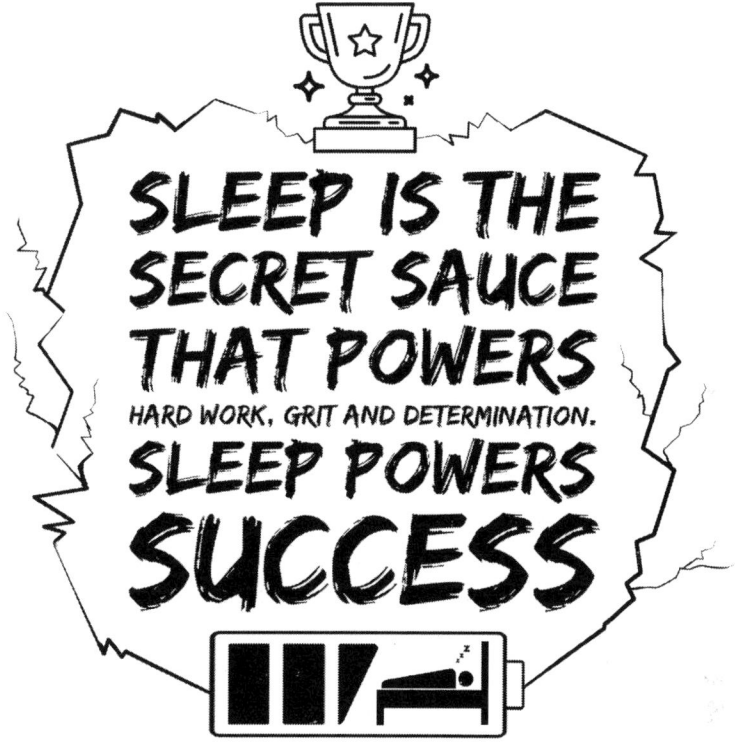

Sleep? I thought you would say hard work, grit and determination—I hear you say.

Ah—but sleep is the secret sauce that powers hard work, grit and determination.

Sleep powers Success!

Good Night!

Goal Sculpting

If you did the Pizza of Life process, you will have at least three essays written out by you about how you want your life to that you want to achieve and who you want to become and why.

This exercise can take some people on flights of fantasy where they create an impossible utopian vision. Others may create something that is way too mundane and simplistic. Both have failure built into them.

Comfort Zone

I was running a volunteers' meeting to organise a fundraiser concert for one of Art of Living's social initiatives. After all the planning and strategising, the key thing for the success of the event that needed to be done boiled down to selling tickets.

We had around 100 volunteers in the room. We planned to do an event with around 1500 participating, meaning we needed to sell 1500 tickets to get the requisite butts in the seats. I am a great believer in the strength of numbers. As the Sanskrit proverb goes—*Sanghe shakti kali yuge*—in these times of the Kali Yuga (difficult times), success will come to those who band together and work towards a common goal.

I said this to them and asked a simple question, 'How many tickets will you personally sell for the event?'

I told people to be honest with the answer. We passed around pieces of paper and asked them to write on it the number of tickets they would individually sell. I said to them, whatever number you write, you promise you will do it and you will move heaven and earth to guarantee it happens. I recognised that there were some people who wouldn't be able to sell even a single ticket because they had other jobs to do. And I mentioned that a zero would be acceptable too. They were not to write their names on the bits of paper. Just the number of tickets they would sell. It was for us as a group to figure out where we were, and therefore how our future plans would need to be created.

People wrote out numbers ranging from 0 to 20. We reached a total of 400-odd tickets that the volunteers in the room promised they would sell.

I knew the people in the room were capable of much, much more—double at least, if not more.

I asked them what my original question to them was.

People shouted it out, 'How many tickets will you personally sell for the event?'

I asked them what they answered and many shouted out their number. I asked them again what they had answered and still quite a few shouted out the number they had written. I asked the question to them 7-8 times till they grew quiet and started thinking …

I gently said, 'I asked you how many tickets you will personally sell. I told you that whatever number you write you will guarantee that come what may, you would sell those many tickets.

'As I said this, almost all of you sat and did some mental math. Then you wrote a number on the piece of paper, and I think most of you wrote a wrong answer.'

Dead silence in the room. I paused for effect …

'The number you gave me was not the answer to my question. I didn't ask you how many tickets you would *comfortably* sell. I asked you how many tickets you *would* sell. I didn't mention anything about comfort in that question. Yet, isn't the answer you gave me something to do with your comfort levels?'

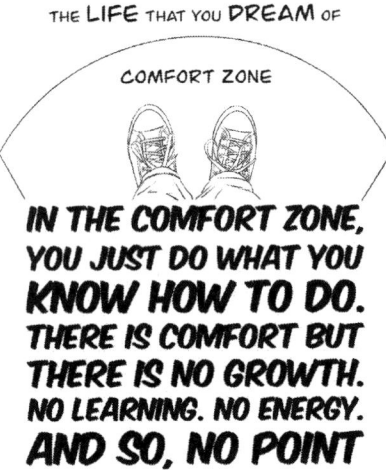

What's the point of doing something you are comfortable doing? The fact that you are comfortable doing it means you know how to do it and it's just a question of execution. Is there any growth? Any stretch? Any learning at all?

In the comfort zone, you just do what you know how to do. There is comfort but there is no growth. No learning. No energy. And so, according to me—no point.

Courage Zone

I invited them to step into their Courage Zone.

A courage zone target is when you *know* you will make it happen, but you have no idea how. Thinking about such a target brings a lump to your throat as you swallow. It makes your heart beat faster. It empowers you and spurs you into action. It awakens, inspires and energises you and the people around you.

When you operate in the courage zone, there is a distinct possibility of failure. You are taking calculated risks. The rewards are far greater as well … and the fact that you had no idea how you were going to accomplish that target means that in the implementation you will learn valuable life lessons and skill up yourself to take on even bigger challenges.

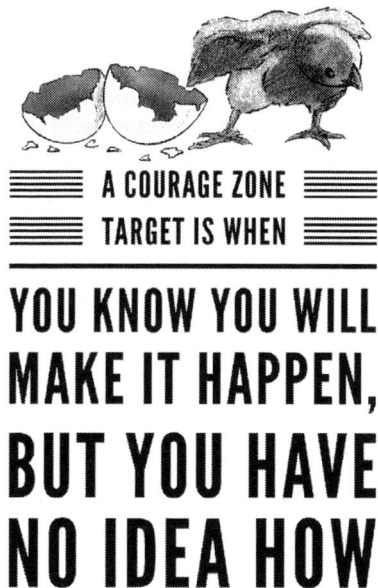

A COURAGE ZONE TARGET IS WHEN YOU KNOW YOU WILL MAKE IT HAPPEN, BUT YOU HAVE NO IDEA HOW

They all became quite kicked and enthusiastic as they heard this. We passed the pieces of paper around again and had them write the number of tickets they would sell—not comfortably sell.

I reminded them to write their courage zone target …

This time, the numbers added up to more than 4000.

Many of them in the heat of the moment had overcommitted.

Overwhelm Zone

I congratulated them and they all cheered when they heard that their projected numbers had jumped from 600 to over 4000. Then as the applause died down, I invited them to think again.

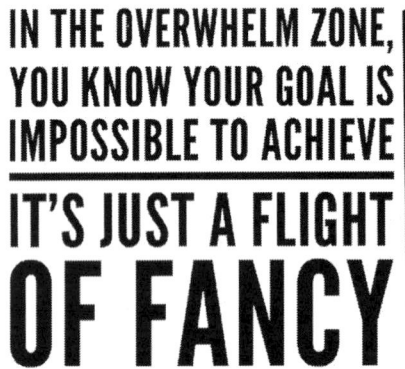
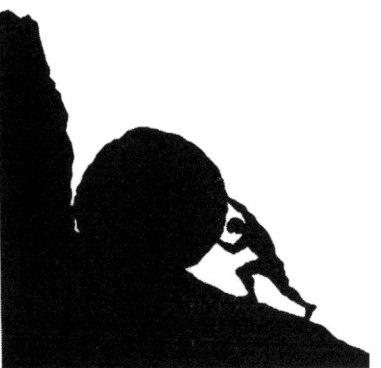

I asked you to get into the courage zone—not the overwhelm zone. I drew the diagram below.

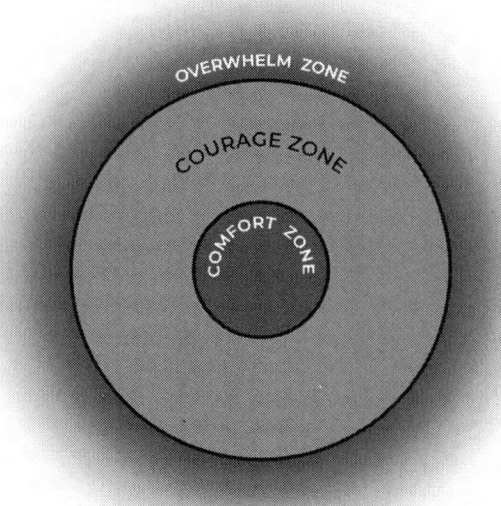

Comfort zone = you know you can do it.

Courage zone = you know you can do it. You just don't know how.

Overwhelm zone = you know you actually cannot do it. You simply got carried away. Your target is not rooted in reality. It is fantasy.

It is easy to stay in the comfort zone and equally easy in a burst of misplaced enthusiasm to leap into the overwhelm zone. The skill is to operate from the courage zone.

I didn't need to pass out papers yet again.

Our event was a grand success. More than 2000 people enjoyed the show, and after all expenses, we had managed to raise more money for the cause than we thought we would.

Take a long hard look at your essays from the Pizza of Life. Are they comfort zone essays? Or have you overwhelmed yourself by setting yourself up to be a victim of an overactive imagination?

Sculpt your essays to bring you squarely into the courage zone. Take a bit of time to think this through. You will know you are there when you wake up each morning with anticipation and enthusiasm about life, raring to go and make a difference to your life and to the lives of people around you.

Trap

Having said all this, there are a few people who will overthink their goals. They will meticulously want to plan out each and every detail before they start working towards their dreams. They will do all sorts of scrutiny and exploration before they even think about getting down to action. They need all their t's crossed and i's dotted. They just plan, plan, plan and never get into actual action. They live in their heads and become the fatalities of Analysis Paralysis.

Fall into this trap and you will end up getting ensnared in just planning and dreaming. Plans are great, but it's action that creates reality. Don't use planning as an excuse to procrastinate.

As you sculpt your goals, give yourself a definite planning timeline by the end of which you will jump into action. You have to realise that goal setting is almost always a work in progress, and its progress is determined by your actions, not just by thinking. As life unfolds, the best laid out plans may need to be abandoned or modified because of the dictates of reality. Oftentimes you may require to be agile and versatile. Being ready for this is intelligence.

Make plans. Have goals. This gives you direction and focuses your energy. But don't take too long. Start moving towards them. It is said that time itself will eat the fruits of delayed action. Don't allow that to happen. Make time your friend.

Don't be in a hurry to get into action. Give yourself the luxury of time to create your essays from the Pizza of Life. Action without strategy is the noise before failure.

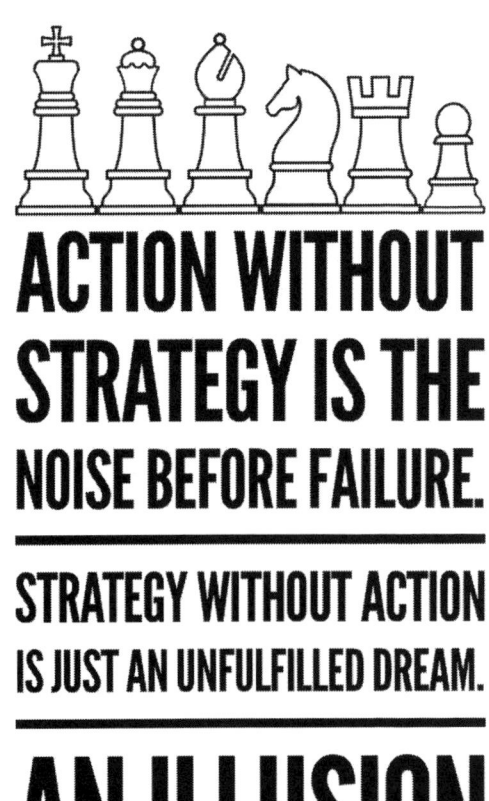

ACTION WITHOUT STRATEGY IS THE NOISE BEFORE FAILURE.

STRATEGY WITHOUT ACTION IS JUST AN UNFULFILLED DREAM.

AN ILLUSION

At the same time, it is critical to set a deadline to finish the planning and ensure that you do get into action. And soon. Strategy without action is just an unfulfilled dream. An illusion.

When will you finish your planning and get into action?

> Write the date here: _____

Get a pen and write the date. Do it!
Good Night!

Superpowers

My friend Gowri has an incredible physique. He is not one of those walking hunks of meat with huge biceps, a gargantuan chest and an enormous back. Rather, he is perfectly proportioned with exactly the right amounts of bulges in exactly the right places. He has that perfect V shape and astounding strength, flexibility and energy.

He hardly needs to do anything to maintain his body. Of course, he exercises, but he does it twice or thrice a week, and not with too much intensity. He just glides and floats around his house using more or less his body weight, and hardly any equipment, many times, having a conversation with anyone who happens to be around.

Yes, he has a great diet. He is vegan and eats fruits and vegetables and avoids sugar and refined flour, but he is open to eating junk now and then.

For him, it is utterly simple to keep his body in amazing shape. His physique is his superpower. Late one night, we were chatting about this and stumbled upon a realisation. He has spent a lifetime being athletic. He totally enjoys yoga and meditation, and has been practising for over a decade. Genetics definitely gave him a push in the right direction, but his unwavering commitment to his health and fitness was what clinched the deal.

Now his body is so well-tuned, he doesn't have to do much to keep it in awesome physical condition.

For me, it's writing. Give me a topic, and I can magically belt out amazing content in a jiffy. I realised I have always enjoyed writing. And so I did a lot of it. Even in school, English was my most favourite subject. I remember an extremely strict English teacher called me to the staff room one afternoon. She handed me an essay I had written with an 8/10 scribbled on the top. She smiled and told me that this was the highest marks she had ever given anyone in her entire career as a teacher, and patted me on my back for a job well done.

I shyly asked her why she had not given me a 10/10. Her eyes twinkled as she said, 'Oh, then you would have to be Shakespeare!'

Over the years, I wrote and wrote and wrote. This has made me become effortlessly good at it. Just like Gowri doesn't need to exercise every single day and keep a calorie count on what he eats, I don't really need to write every single day to stay in touch. Whenever I need to, it just flows. Writing is my superpower.

Dr Ankita Dhelia is a gifted healer. Though she trained conventionally to become a doctor, she found her true calling through alternative healing modalities. Over the years, she has deeply studied Osteopathy, Craniosacral Therapy, NeuroKinetic Therapy, the Bach Flower remedies, Naturopathy etc. deeply.

The result? She just has to put her hands on someone, and in a few minutes she can read that person. She can tell them what's wrong with them, what and where their pain or discomfort is and what they can do to fix it.

She uses the vast knowledge that she has accumulated about the human body to non-invasively help a person who may have been recommended surgery, bringing them back to health. She has saved hundreds of people from the surgeon's knife, sparing them the pain and trauma of an operation, not to mention the huge financial burden that would be inevitable.

Her superpower is healing.

Harshal doesn't just sing like an angel. Angels come to him for singing lessons!

In a concert hall, he lights up the stage and transports the audience to an alternate reality on wings of his songs. For him, practising music and singing are as natural as breathing. And he has been doing that for over two decades.

The finesse, maturity and expression in his voice are a testament to his dedication to music. So now it's easy and seemingly effortless.

His superpower is singing.

While I was writing this chapter, I got on a phone call with a dear friend and she asked me what I was doing. So I described to her all about this chapter and she said, 'But I don't have any superpower.'

I know she is brilliant at networking. She has an incredibly wide social network comprising of some of the most successful people I know. People connect with her easily, and she has the ability to make almost anyone feel at ease. This is precisely her superpower. When I told her all this, she responded with a surprised, 'Really?!'

It was then that I realised we all seem to take our superpowers for granted. Gowri feels his awesome physique is not a big deal. Harshal doesn't think too highly of his exquisite singing. I feel that writing is so easy, anyone can do it.

Our superpowers are a case of simplicity on the far, far side of complexity.

Because these powers are so much a part of us, we become dismissive of them. We say they are a gift, or it's just genetics. We don't acknowledge that we have truly invested a lot to develop them.

This is the reason most of us don't end up strategically using these powers to our advantage. We don't harness them to get us to where we truly want to get to in life. We get trapped in middle-class monotony. Our dreams remain dreams.

What's your superpower?

How do you use it to align your actions towards what you want to manifest in your life?

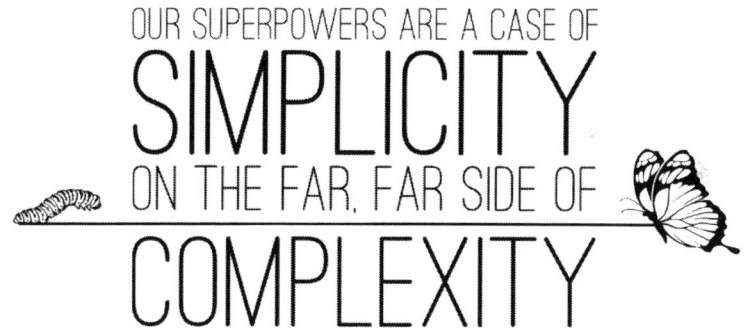

OUR SUPERPOWERS ARE A CASE OF
SIMPLICITY
ON THE FAR, FAR SIDE OF
COMPLEXITY

The Expertise Trap

In my twenties, I had developed a keen interest in western classical music. My two big sources of listening to this music were the British Council Library and the National Centre for the Performing Arts—both located at least an hour away from where I lived in Mumbai.

Though it was quite an effort to get there, I would go to both these places as often as I could and spend many hours listening to the wondrous music created by the masters who had lived more than two or three centuries before I was born. A lot of this music had beautiful melodies and I would hum them throughout the day—an orchestra playing solely for me in my head.

If you wanted to truly appreciate the classics, you would need to listen to them over and over again to notice the subtleties—a little flute passage here, an exquisite horn solo there, the sudden boom of a kettle drum, the delicate tinkling of a triangle, an effortlessly dramatic change in key. These little nuances scattered around the music were the essence of the genius of the masters. The glorious magic of the classics was brought to life by these gorgeous little passages.

I found the popular music of the day tedious, repetitive and bland and could never understand how other people seemed to enjoy it. I dare say I became quite a music snob.

I relish the classics even today. But many times, these days, I feel listening to them is just too much work. While I do listen to some Tchaikovsky, Chopin or Liszt, after a while I find myself wanting something easy to enjoy. I then move to some pop and even manage to enjoy it for a bit—but soon I find it too trite and flavourless, and switch it off.

I found that this pattern repeats in different aspects of my life. I love playing board games, but they are too much trouble to set up and explain to others. It is easier to play something quick on my iPad. I love cooking and eating great food—but unless there is someone coming over, it's easier to settle for some simple dal and veggies. I love to exercise when I have a trainer with me—but when I am alone, I find myself preferring to take a long walk instead of going through the grind of push-ups, squats and lunges.

I could go on, but you get the idea.

Does this resonate with you as well? Have you ever thought about what was going on, and why this happened?

According to me, there are two reasons why this happens.

Focus

There is a question I get asked all the time when I teach meditation courses.

I get bored easily, how do I focus? I can't seem to concentrate at all.

This seems to have become the bane for so many people—they cannot focus even when they want to. Even when they are interested. This inability to focus develops because of what we are doing when we are not doing the stuff we need to focus on.

Throughout the day we are on digital messenger apps or on social media. We incessantly surf channels on our TV. What we are unconsciously doing is training our brain to pay attention for just a few seconds. Over and over and over again. And we have been doing this for an appreciably long time. For the younger generations, this is all they have been doing since as far back as they can remember.

When something important comes up and you need to be able to focus, you simply cannot. You have trained your brain differently.

Solution: Be careful about what you are doing throughout the day. Your brain is like an innocent child—it will learn, and learn well. Be careful about what you teach it. The good news is that it is quite elastic and can unlearn and relearn as well. In your free time, ensure you are creating the brain you want, so that when it's time to work, your physiology cooperates with you.

I am pretty sure that social media and my consumption of it has made me impatient with classical music. Pop music gives me that quick fix that I was looking for. Unfortunately, pop lacks the depth and sheer beauty of the classics. When I take a break from the buzz of information that I allow myself to be bombarded with, my ability to enjoy the classics gets rekindled.

You are in control of how much exposure you want to give to brain-numbing activity. Dance with the dopamine, don't give into its allure (for more about dopamine, read the chapter 'Dancing with Dopamine').

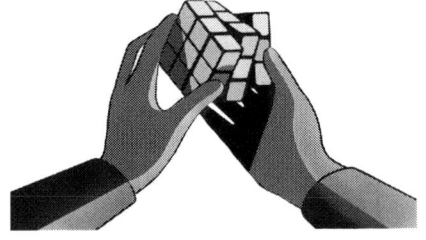

THE INABILITY TO FOCUS **DEVELOPS BECAUSE OF** WHAT WE ARE DOING, WHEN WE ARE NOT DOING THE STUFF WE NEED TO FOCUS ON

Boredom

When something piques our interest, we give a lot of ourselves to it. If it is something that we really want to achieve and is in our courage zone, we devote a lot of time and energy to it. We research, learn and practice until we become reasonably good at it.

At the point we consider ourselves an expert on it, it moves out of our courage zone and into our comfort zone. It no longer challenges us as it did before. We reach a peak, only to find a plateau there. It is easy to get stuck on this plateau.

A friend of mine, an ardent lover of Hindustani classical music, used to go to his Guru to learn singing. His Guru would make him sing the notes 'Sa re ga ma pa dha ni sa' over and over and over again for months on end. Once, out of frustration he burst out saying, 'I know the notes. I am bored of singing the same thing again and again for so many months. Can you please teach me something more?'

The Guru smiled and gently replied, 'You know the notes? After all these years, I am still trying to get Sa right!'

When you think you know, and consider yourself an expert, boredom sets in. You make it all right for yourself to be on the plateau of your peak. However, to reach the pinnacle of true perfection, to become a master, requires great humility, dedication and faith. Humility, to acknowledge that there is a colossal amount of knowledge still left to learn and explore. Dedication, to keep going despite not being able to see conspicuous improvements. Faith, that your practice will eventually bear fruit.

Boredom comes from repetition. You have to do the same thing again and again, day after day, for months or years on end, barely seeing any noticeable development. You wonder about the point of it. And mostly, you stop ... choosing the plateau over the pinnacle.

This is actually all right when it comes to the more pedestrian aspects of life. You don't need to spend time and effort brewing a better cup of tea. Or creating even more delicious pasta. Or making your bed to perfection. Or tying your shoe laces faster. Expertise in these cases is often more than enough.

However, for things that really matter to you in life, boredom can create an unsurmountable barrier between expertise and mastery.

Mastery

Everyone knows that meditation dramatically improves one's quality of life. People start off on their spiritual journey with

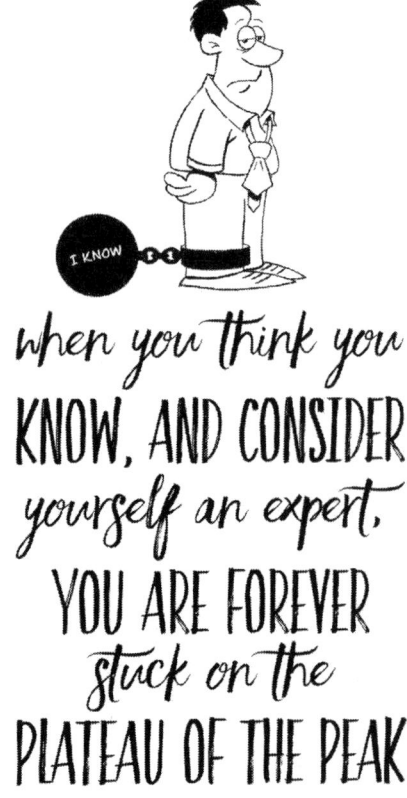

when you think you KNOW, AND CONSIDER yourself an expert, YOU ARE FOREVER stuck on the PLATEAU OF THE PEAK great enthusiasm as they see vast quality of life improvements as they practice. In a while, they begin to consider themselves expert meditators.

Unfortunately, as time passes, they stop seeing the big changes. There will be minuscule changes that will add up over time, but in themselves seem almost irrelevant. Most often these changes may even go unobserved. This is when people start feeling bored, and either slip up on their practice or go on a spiritual shopping spree finding more techniques so they can do something different.

This, in turn, will create a gradual deterioration in their expertise ... as this happens, they begin to slip up even more in their practice, feeling that it's not helping them anymore. This downward spiral can bring even long-term meditators almost back to where they were when they first began to meditate.

Replace meditation with anything you consider worth achieving in life and you will know exactly what I mean. You could be an expert cook but boredom might have stopped you short of becoming a masterchef. You could be an expert on the stock market, but boredom might have denied you mastery. You could be a brilliant manager, but the boredom of dealing with the sameness of your job might have stopped you from becoming the CEO. You may be a great athlete, but boredom will impede you from winning an Olympic gold.

Many people become millionaires. Very few become billionaires.

People become victims of the boredom trap. Humility, dedication and faith all go for a toss.

The obvious question then is, 'How do I take off from the plateau of expertise to soar into the sky of mastery?'

There is no easy way.

Maharishi Patanjali, in his *Yoga Sutras*, says:
'Sa tu Deergha Kaala
Nairantarya
Satkaara Sevitoh
Dridha Bhoomi'

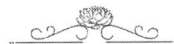

स तु दीर्घकाल नैरन्तर्यसत्कारासेवितो
दृढभूमिः ॥

Freely translated, this means:

'When you do something for a long, long time, without a break, with reverence and honour for it, only then will you get established in the practice of it.'

You start as a beginner and with practice become a novice. Determination and grit will transform you into an expert. If you can still manage to faithfully continue your practice with the zeal and humility of a beginner, for a long, long time, then, in time, you will achieve mastery.

This is how millions turn into billions.

And what is Mastery?

Mastery means making it look simple and obvious to the ones who are watching. So simple that everyone feels even they could do it; that it's no big deal.

A Master of the Martial Arts had once said, 'When you begin to learn martial arts, a punch is a punch and a kick is a kick. As you progress towards expertise, you understand the complexity and the art behind each move. A punch is not just a punch—it's so much more. A kick is not just a kick—there is such beauty in the intricacy of the movement. But once you attain mastery, a punch is a punch and a kick is a kick.'

Mastery is simplicity on the far side of complexity.
What do you wish to master in your life?
Persevere, and eventually you will get there.
Good Night!

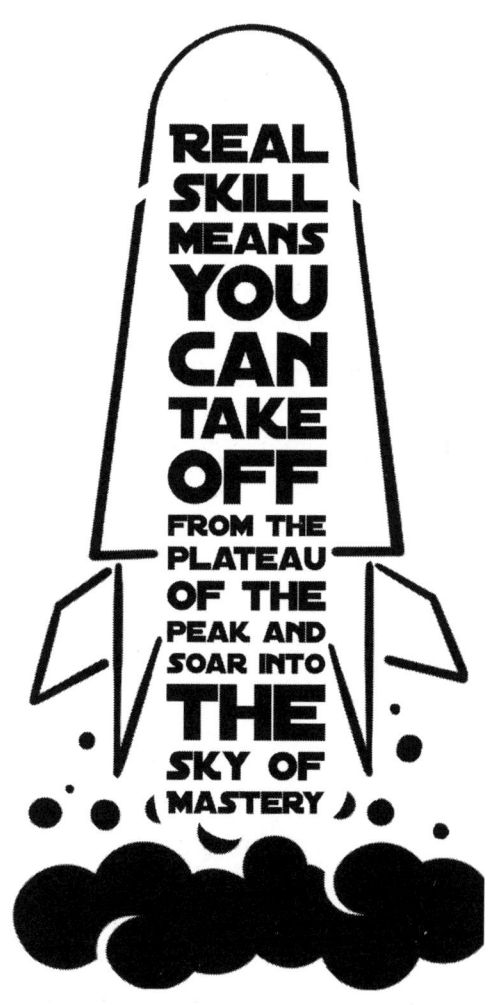

Lines

Starting in late 2019, Covid-19, a highly infectious strain of the flu virus (SARS type), has infected approximately 37 million people around the world as I write this. More than a million people have succumbed to it.

One individual Coronavirus (that caused Covid-19) weighs 0.85 attogram—that's 0.00000000000000000085 gm. To give you an idea about exactly how small that is, take something that weighs 0.85 gm, then divide that into one million parts. Now take one of those parts and divide that into ten million sections. One part from this is the weight of a Coronavirus—0.85 attogram.

Less than just 20 gm of the insidious Coronavirus brought life as we knew it on planet Earth to a grinding halt.

The only way to curtail the spread of this virus was to enforce a complete worldwide lockdown. People couldn't step out of their homes, except for essential goods. Shopping malls, stadiums, schools and colleges, offices, movie theatres and all other places where people would gather were shut down for a few months. The Olympics were postponed. There was no national or international travel. Airlines the world over grounded their planes.

A fever meant panic. Self-isolation, social distancing, wearing masks and face shields became common practice. All over the world, doctors and scientists fought valiantly to save as many lives as possible. And to their credit, they mostly succeeded.

The impact that this virus had even on people not affected by it at all was humungous. Daily wage workers were the hardest hit—there was no work and so no money for them, and many faced starvation. Millions of people helped NGOs and governments step in to ensure these poor people had enough to eat and to survive. Hundreds of thousands of people lost their jobs. Scores of businesses declared bankruptcy. The economic devastation was in billions of dollars.

Not everything was grim, though. As travel was completely restricted and city roads went quiet, the sounds of nature filtered through. Dolphins were sighted in the seas near the beaches in Mumbai. Some rare species of animals made appearances. The air became cleaner as the dust of pollution settled. The waters of rivers the world over became clearer and fish not seen in decades were spotted. Humanity in quarantine made Mother Nature rejoice.

Dinesh and I were fortunate to spend the quarantine on our pristine Art of Living ashram in Bangalore and were spared much of the horror. Our community at the ashram, too, had quite a scare as one single case multiplied to a few dozen in a week's time. Apart from one person who died of a heart attack, everyone else recovered completely.

Throughout the pandemic, friends from all over the world would call and tell us about what would be going on in their lives, how they were coping. We heard many fascinating stories—of despair and courage, of hope, of love and of loss.

Psychologically, entire swathes of the population were deeply affected. Many couldn't deal with the enforced isolation, and developed all sorts of mental and domestic issues. Many couples who thought they were in love with each other discovered they couldn't stand each other. Others on the verge of divorce discovered love all over again. Families broke up or came even closer together.

The true colours of people stood harshly revealed.

As we heard hundreds of stories of people coping or breaking, Dinesh and I started to see a sort of pattern emerge. A vast majority of the people we knew who coped, even thrived, during this challenging time had a strong sense of who they were, what they needed to do and what they were worth.

They were the ones who knew how to draw the line. Let me explain.

A friend of mine, Trupti, a brilliant creative designer, was one of the first people we know who lost her job. She was earning close to Rs 1.5 lakh a month. As advertising agencies were shutting down in the wake of the Coronavirus pandemic, there were simply no jobs available. She had some savings and managed for a while, but was quickly going into the red zone as days passed and no one wanted to hire her.

One day, she called me in desperation. She sobbed as she told me her story. A few months ago, there were projects lined up for her, and she had had to say no. Now there was just no work. What could she do? I told her to pray and keep trying.

Three days later, she called again. She had landed a job that was paying her just Rs 30,000 a month. She was in a huge dilemma whether to accept or not. It was clearly demeaning for her to work for that paltry sum. She didn't want to do it. Yet, Rs 30,000 was better than nothing.

She knew I coached people and asked me for a one-on-one session. I had been wanting a really nice logo design done for a long time and agreed to barter a coaching session or two for the logo and layouts for my website.

I started by asking her about the absolute minimum salary she was ready to work for. What was the value she attributed to her work and herself? She hummed and haahed and said she would want Rs 1.5 lakh a month, but would settle for Rs 1 lakh a month. I asked her again if she would be willing to work for less than a lakh a month. She said no … but there was not much conviction in the no.

We went deeper into the question and explored her relationship with money, her self worth and other related topics, until she had completely convinced herself that Rs 1 lakh a month was the bare minimum she would accept as compensation for her work.

Then I asked her about her original dilemma—whether she wanted to accept that job at Rs 30,000 a month—and this time, with full conviction she said no way.

I asked her if she would take up an offer of Rs 75,000 a month and again she said no. And what about Rs 99,999 a month? Would she take that? She understood where I was taking her and smiled and confidently said no. She had drawn a line—Rs 1 lakh or not at all.

She was ready to move to the next level.

When I coach people, one of the things I do is open them to possibilities they could almost never figure out by themselves. I asked her another question, 'If there was no way you could land a job as a designer, what would you do? Assume it's just impossible to earn any money from designing. Now what?!'

Her eyes opened wide. This possibility had just not occurred to her. She had been so busy looking for a job, and so disappointed that she had not found one, that she had not considered anything else.

She sat back in her chair and told me, 'Did you know I love baking? I make the most amazing cakes. Maybe I could sell them? But who would buy them from me?'

Covid or no Covid, there are going to be birthdays and anniversaries. Cakes are going to be required. And people would rather buy a cake from a known person than a shop, given the concerns about hygiene. I told her all this and reminded her that she was a designer and there was something called Instagram.

She didn't need a second call with me.

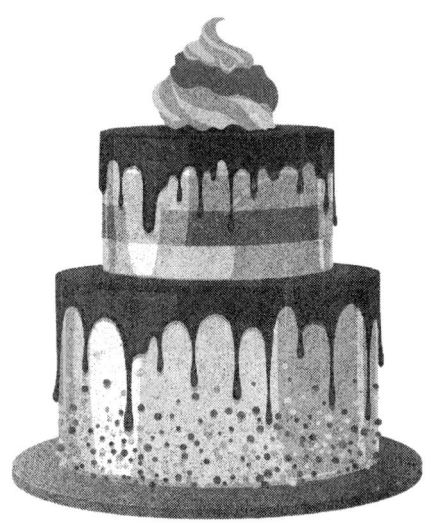

She went to work with gusto, designed a fabulous logo and brand name and went public on Instagram (@justcakeit_bakery). Slowly, orders started trickling in. Her customers enjoyed her cakes and talked about them to their friends and families. As the word spread, more and more people e-queued up to buy them. In October, she sold enough cakes to actually earn her more than what she was being paid as a designer in her earlier job.

She called me a few days back, totally ecstatic. She was wondering if she should go 'artisanal' or start a whole chain of stores that produced baked goodies. As the lockdown was being lifted and some semblance of normalcy was being established, some companies were approaching her and offering her designer jobs. It was easy for her to say no to them and tell them instead that she would work on a project-to-project basis as a freelancer.

She quipped that she wouldn't work for free, though—she would be quite expensive.

She had drawn lines and stayed above them. She now knew when to say no. She could recognise when a door was closed to her and not waste precious time and energy trying to pry it open. She could move on, looking for other doors and other opportunities.

When you draw the line somewhere, it gives you a sense of identity. Your line tells you who you are and makes it very easy for you to decide when to say yes and when to say no.

I am a vegetarian. All non-vegetarian food is strictly no-no for me. There is no way I am going to eat any of that stuff.

I was talking about drawing the line to a bunch of students and when I said this, one guy says, 'But if I am stuck in a jungle and have only non-veg food to eat to survive, then what?'

What is the probability of you ever getting into a situation like that? You might as well ask what if you are stuck on the moon. Or on Tatooine. Or Middle Earth—J.R.R. Tolkien land. These are all fantasies and hypothetical situations. Often you fool yourself into not drawing lines and compromising on your ideals by thinking like this.

So yes, I am a vegetarian and I don't eat any non-veg food at all. This is a line I have drawn for myself. Once I was on a twelve-hour flight and they didn't have any vegetarian food on board. I was starving. Did I eat the chicken curry? Absolutely not. That was simply not acceptable to me. It was way below my line.

When I politely explained this to the crew, they made me a hot chocolate drink and gave me some bread, butter, cheese and jam. And a big platter of fruits. If my line was not firmly drawn, hunger might have made me compromise.

Where are your lines on various aspects of your life, and have you drawn them firmly enough? Would you be willing to compromise on your ideals? What would make you do that? What will you simply not compromise on? What kind of character do you have? Who are the people you are willing to call your friends? What is your relationship with money? Who will you do business with?

These are interesting questions to ponder upon as they bring clarity about who you are. When you know who you are, it's just easier to make choices.

When there is a choice between right and wrong, almost everyone will choose right.

The conundrum is when you have to make a choice between right and convenient. Choosing convenient is easier than choosing right, in that moment. But choosing right ultimately brings you a sense of peace and dramatically boosts your self esteem. When your lines are hazy, and life becomes challenging, you usually end up doing what's convenient—and regret that decision for a long, long time.

Be especially wary of the stuff that's just below your line. Develop a habit of keeping what's below the line, below the line. Even when it's *just* below the line. Clearly defined lines mean that you have a strong sense of identity and you will consistently choose right over convenient.

Do this, and for sure you will sleep better.
Good Night!

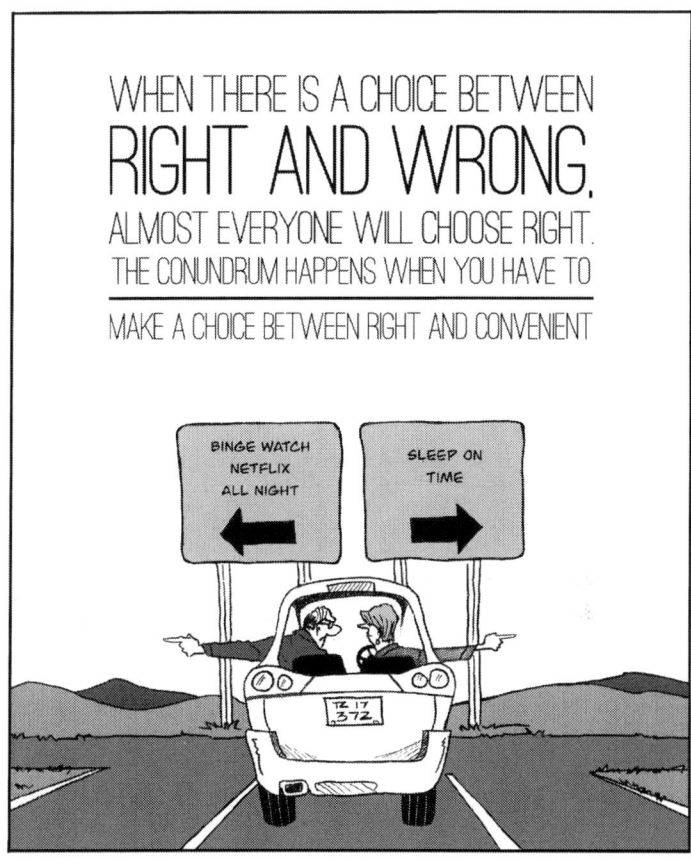

Letting Go

There is a part of your mind that is quite strange. It doesn't like letting go of people or situations even when those people or situations are actively making you miserable. You may have invested a lot of time, money and effort and simply because of this, your mind keeps telling you it has to get better. It will get better. It cannot deteriorate any further. And you continue to hang on, feeling worse each passing day, just refusing to let go. A simple example would be a movie you pay Rs 200 to watch. You get into the theatre, the movie starts ... and it sucks. Yet, most people would sit and watch the entire thing till the end—somewhere secretly hoping it would end well, or pick up pace, or have a really funny scene, or something else that would make it worth your while. You don't like the movie—it's boring and you and you are hating the experience—why are you still sitting through it? The director, producer and actors are not paying you to watch the movie. In fact, you actually paid them. If it's bad, the obvious thing to do would be to get up, get out and do something else!

But you don't. Woody Allen starts his movie *Annie Hall* with a little anecdote that he narrates:

Two little old women are sitting at a restaurant eating food.

One says to the other, 'The food here is terrible!'

The other nods and replies, 'Yes, and the portions are so small too.'

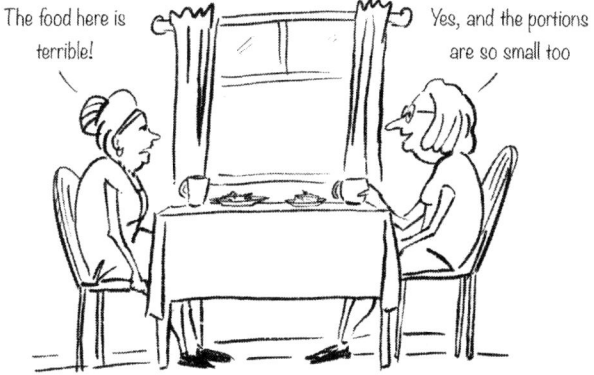

The Grandfather

One of our elder Swamijis from Art of Living used to go and stay with a family up in Uttarakhand which comprised of an old man, his son, the son's wife and their two kids who were brats. The old man would take care of the kids, cook the food, do the dishes, clean the house, wash and even iron the clothes.

There wasn't an iota of gratitude from the family for what the old man did. They would order him about and frequently even abuse him. The old man's eyes would sometimes tear up, but no one would even notice, let alone bother to apologise. There was never a word of appreciation. Only orders were barked at him all day, and many times late into the night.

Our Swamiji's heart melted at this unforgivably harsh treatment meted out to the grandfather, and one day he told the old man, 'Come away with me. I have a nice place in the ashram. You can stay with me. You don't need to go through this abuse …'

Before Swamiji could even finish the sentence, the old man got offended and angry and shouted, 'If I come with you, who will cook? Who will take care of my grandchildren? Who will clean the house? You are trying to break up my family. You call yourself spiritual? You should be ashamed!'

Swamiji was flabbergasted. Here was a person choosing to be abused—choosing to stay in a living hell, all because of that weird attachment to 'family'. He shook his head and left the old man to the misery he had wilfully chosen.

This is an extreme example of not being able to let go and move on—of the mind actually making it feel alright to be abused, day in and day out.

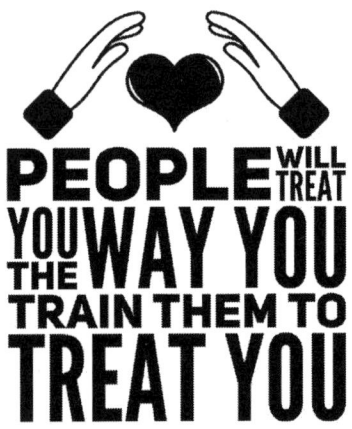

Now think about your life.

Translate all this into what's not working in your life—why do you still have that parasite of a friend? Or that business that your grandfather started eighty years ago, that's been steadily making a loss and showing no signs that it will ever improve? Or that secretary who has been with you for years and was inefficient and a headache from the first month? Or those shares you bought at Rs 600 which are now worth Rs 50, with no hope of them ever going up?

Why are you not getting up and getting out?! What's stopping you?

Boozing

When I was studying in IITB, I had a bunch of dear friends. We liked each other a lot and hung out together—mostly we got drunk together. Every weekend. In retrospect, more than anything, I think it was the booze that kept us together. The booze was a kind of a lifeline and helped me deal with the pressure. I feel booze allowed me to remain sane in the cutthroat competitive environment that was IITB. It was the only way I knew at that time.

Then I did the Art of Living course and learned to meditate. I found I could relax my mind at will and deal with the inevitable stress of studying in one of India's best educational institutions. I definitely didn't need that alcohol coursing through my system any more. I was excited and told all my friends about it. I was taken aback when they refused to learn meditation, preferring to stay with the bottle.

Very soon, as my system became more and more refined, I started to find their company repulsive. The indiscipline, the bad breath, the abusive language, the whining and the vomiting after a night of getting drunk could not be a part of my life anymore. I started to drift away from these people. But they were not willing to let me go so easily. They would taunt me, tease me … calling me all sorts of names, saying I had given up on years of friendship—all for some silly meditation.

For me, it was no longer friendship. It was delusion. And it had been a long spell of delusion. Years of it. Thankfully, as realisation dawned, I was intelligent enough to let go of these people and get out of their lives. I was brave enough to move on.

As this happened, the truly special people got a chance to enter my life. Dinesh was one of them.

It may be true that you may have invested a great deal in something, but at some point, you may need to make a decision to start saying a vehement no. Because it's simply not worth it any more.

However much your mind rebels, have the courage to say no.

People will treat you the way you train them to treat you.

The Dog

There was this man who went to stay at a farmhouse in the countryside. It was beautiful and peaceful and serene and he enjoyed his first day. At night, something peculiar happened. The neighbour's dog started to howl mournfully and then cried out in pain. And the howling went on and on for a few hours. The man was tired that night, so didn't pay too much attention. The next night it happened again. And then again and again, and it went on every single night for a week.

At first the man felt it was none of his business. Then he couldn't stand the thought of that poor animal in pain each and every night, and decided to go talk to the neighbour about it.

He went over to the farm next door and was welcomed in by a grizzled old woman.

After exchanging the usual pleasantries, the man enquired about the dog. He asked why the animal was in such pain every night. She grunted and took him around to show the dog's kennel. She pointed to a nail and a splinter that was jutting out. She said whenever the dog got into the kennel to sleep at night, the nail hurt him and he howled until he eventually fell asleep.

The man was astonished.

If it hurt the dog, why didn't it move and go someplace else to sleep?

The old woman smiled ruefully as she said, 'It doesn't hurt him enough.'

It doesn't hurt him enough! We don't move on because it doesn't hurt enough. Our mind can numb us towards constant pain and we can become okay with it. It's only when we manage to somehow get ourselves out of that pain that we realise how painful it had become. We make up stories to be all right with what shouldn't be all right. We then end up just enduring. We keep watching that movie …

It would be a great idea to start thinking about all the stuff in your life that's hurting you. Start thinking about all that you are going to start saying no to.

Don't stop at thinking, though. Get up and do it. Get up and get out when the movie sucks.

You will need to say no to certain things so that you can do the things you said yes to brilliantly well.

Good Night!

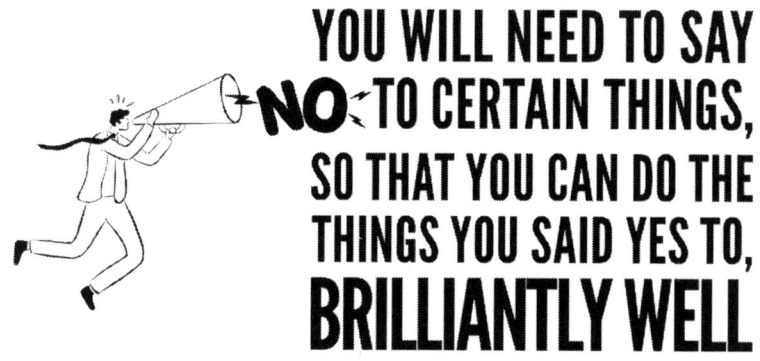

Adding by Subtracting

I am going to let you in on two secrets.

First, we are all intrinsically lazy.

Over the millennia of evolution, our brain has evolved to conserve energy, and so will always look for the quickest and easiest way to get something done. It sounds better when you say it like this. But what it essentially means is that we are hardwired to be lazy.

Secondly, there is a deep desire genetically encoded into us to be happy in the moment. That's not much of a secret … but our brain is programmed to take us towards pleasure and away from pain. Even if pain in the short term creates pleasure in the long term, and pleasure in the short term creates pain in the long term. The brain is all for being delighted right now, and doesn't care much about the consequences of later. It will typically propel you away from action it considers painful, even if those actions will reap rich rewards in the future.

Consider this.

You have decided to have a green smoothie every morning. Green smoothies are nutrition-rich, full of fibre and have truckloads of vitamins and minerals. They contribute towards bone health, better digestion and over time, build a stronger immune system. They even lower cholesterol. You know these smoothies are really good for you. You know they will contribute tremendously to your sense of well-being.

To make a green smoothie, choose two or more of these:
2 celery sticks
A small bunch of spinach
A small bunch of kale
Some watercress leaves
Some microgreens
1 small cucumber
Any green salad leaves

Choose one or more of these:
1 avocado
A small bowl of fresh coconut malai (coconut meat)
1 banana

Choose one or more of these:
1 tsp hemp seeds
1 tsp chia seeds
1 tsp flax seeds

You may add in any of these as well:
1 apple
2 (or more) dates, depending on how sweet you want your smoothie to be
½ inch piece of ginger
1 or 2 pieces of ice

Chop everything and bung it into a powerful mixer grinder. Blend it till smooth. Have it immediately.

If you want to be fancy about it, put the blended greens into a bowl and decorate it with whatever you have on hand—roasted seeds, chopped fresh fruit (pineapple, banana, pomegranate, cherries and apple are delicious and go really well), dried cranberries, raisins, dried mulberries, almond slivers and roasted cashew nuts are all excellent toppings.

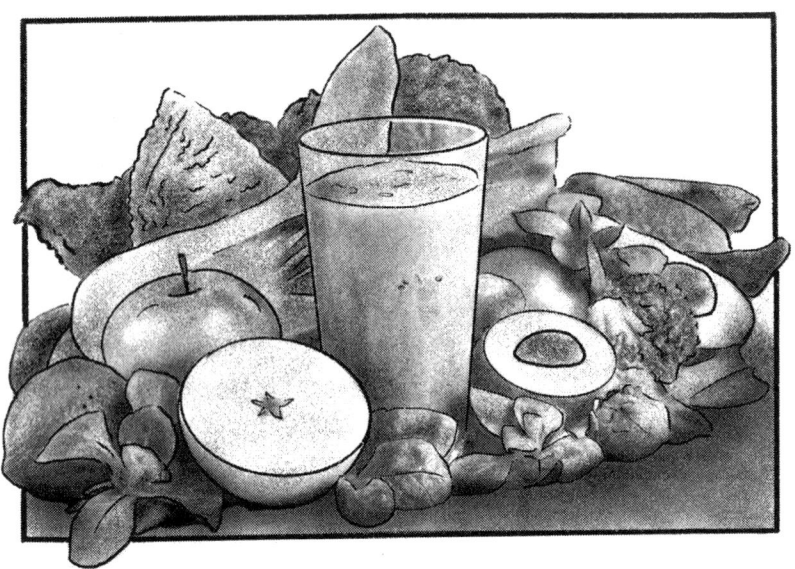

A green smoothie bowl, when made properly, looks gorgeous and tastes delicious.

If you are going to make this from scratch every morning, it's going to take you about 20 minutes, and maybe another 5-10 minutes to clean up and put everything back in its place.

On the other hand, making a cup of tea or coffee is so much simpler and takes less than 5 minutes. A cup of steaming hot tea just feels so much more comforting compared to a cold bowl of pulverised greens early in the morning.

Tea and coffee both have caffeine. Most people also add sugar. And typically, the milk you use will not be reliably sourced organic A2 milk. Did you know that every day India produces 14,000 crore litres of milk, and yet 64,000 crore litres of milk is sold?! The white liquid most people drink thinking it's milk cannot even be considered milk.

The cream you add as a topping for that luxurious five-star feel has a ton of calories.

Just as you know the green smoothie is brilliant for you, you know tea or coffee is not so good for you.

Yet, more often than not, it is tea or coffee that will normally make it to your breakfast table instead of the smoothie. These beverages win because of your brain. They are easy and convenient to make. They give you pleasure in the moment. They check all the boxes as far as your brain is concerned.

Sit back and think of all those 'good-for-you' things you have been wanting to do. You now have some clues about why you didn't do them, or stopped doing them after a while. Either you didn't get immediate pleasure from those activities or they just took up too much time and energy to get done—at least initially.

To build life-enhancing habits, you will need to employ ingenuity to trick your brain. Think of how to make it simple and pleasurable for yourself to do whatever you had decided to do. At the same time, make it inconvenient and painful to do what you don't want to do.

For example, in the case of the green smoothie, prep everything the night before. To discourage yourself from having the tea, lock the sugar in a cupboard that's not in the kitchen and keep the key in your bathroom. When you get to the kitchen in the morning, because everything is chopped and ready, it is that much easier to make the smoothie.

Because the sugar is locked away somewhere, it becomes too much of an effort to make the tea, as compared to the smoothie, and your brain will make you want the smoothie over the tea. Top the smoothie with your favourite toppings and you will have added pleasure into the mix.

Tea or coffee will be history.

Willpower

I loved sweets. My cupboard always had some treats stashed away in case I felt like it.

While researching for our second book, *Happiness Express*, I found out about the terrible consequences of having white sugar.

I decided I would stop having white sugar completely. This meant that, for starters, gulab jamuns, an Indian sweet I adored, were out. Quickly, a realisation dawned—it was not just gulab jamuns—all Indian sweets were out. In fact, all sweets in general were gone from my menu—no cakes, no puddings, no doughnuts, no chocolate, and horror of horrors, no ice cream!

But this was just the beginning. At that time, I had no idea how insidious the usage of sugar is. It is an omnipresent ingredient in almost every commercially available packaged food. This meant that all ketchup, mayonnaise, jams, chutneys and various sauces I used to create delectable meals got tossed into the forbidden list.

I remember how I had once triumphantly found a cooking sauce with no sugar in the ingredients, only to later find out that ethyl maltol, florida crystals, barley malt and sorghum syrup that were on the list of ingredients on that bottle were actually sugar in disguise. With the growing awareness of the horrible effects of white sugar, the big food companies didn't remove it—they just creatively renamed it, hoping that people wouldn't find out their secret. I am sure there are just a handful of nerds like me who would actually google florida crystals to find out exactly what it was.

When I decided I would stop having sugar, I had no idea how incredibly difficult it would be. It was quite a challenge, but I rose up to it. I knew I had tremendous willpower. For about two or three weeks, I was totally off sugar. I righteously said no to the various sweets offered to me and everyone around me was amazed at the change, as they all knew that I had an insatiable sweet tooth.

Then I had a fight with someone dear to me and was feeling really low. The chocolates in my cupboard sang to me. My mind was saying things like—*You are feeling low, you have been brilliant these last few weeks, right now you know that a few pieces of chocolate will make you feel so much better; what harm can two pieces of chocolate do to you?* And so on.

I am sure you know the script of this particular mental dialogue pretty well.

Almost automatically, the chocolates found their way into my mouth ... My willpower had vanished like the morning dew in the heat of the sun.

Willpower takes up a lot of resources to maintain. It's not something the brain likes to exercise. Invariably, willpower will not serve you to consistently keep the promises you make to yourself. You are fighting against millennia of evolution that has programmed your brain to conserve energy, and move you towards what is pleasurable in the moment. At some point you will falter. Inevitably, you will lose.

It is far more intelligent and easier to use evolution to your advantage.

Create an environment that is conducive to what you are aiming towards.

You want to be fit? Hang around with people who are fit—for whom exercise is normal; people who eat healthy. Follow fit and healthy people on your social media. Surround yourself with healthy eating options. Soon, you too will feel the urge to make healthier life choices.

Choose a gym that is easy to get to. On your way to work, for example. If getting to the gym is even a detour of a block or two, it's too much energy wasted to get there, as far as your brain is concerned.

In the first few days of going to the gym, simply workout for five to ten minutes. Not more. You are still keeping this new action as simple as possible. After a week or two, you will begin to feel, *Now that I am here, let me exercise for a few more minutes. Do a few more sets. Build up your habit like this.*

Remember to reward yourself each time you go to the gym and workout. For example, 30 more minutes of playing my favourite video game or senseless scrolling through social media after I worked out were a superb reward for me. The brain then sees that activity as easy and rewarding in the moment. You will find yourself going to the gym more often. In a while, exercise will become part of your routine. Once you feel great because you are exercising, there will be no need for the reward. When this happens, you know that now exercise is part of your identity.

Want to meditate regularly? Choose to be with people who are regular meditators. A friend from IIT who had done the Art of Living course ages ago had never practised what he had learned. He got a new job and moved to Bangalore. His house was near the ashram. Our ashram is a stunningly beautiful place and he took to coming every evening for a walk there. I am pretty sure the pizzas in Café Vishala added to the charm of the place for him.

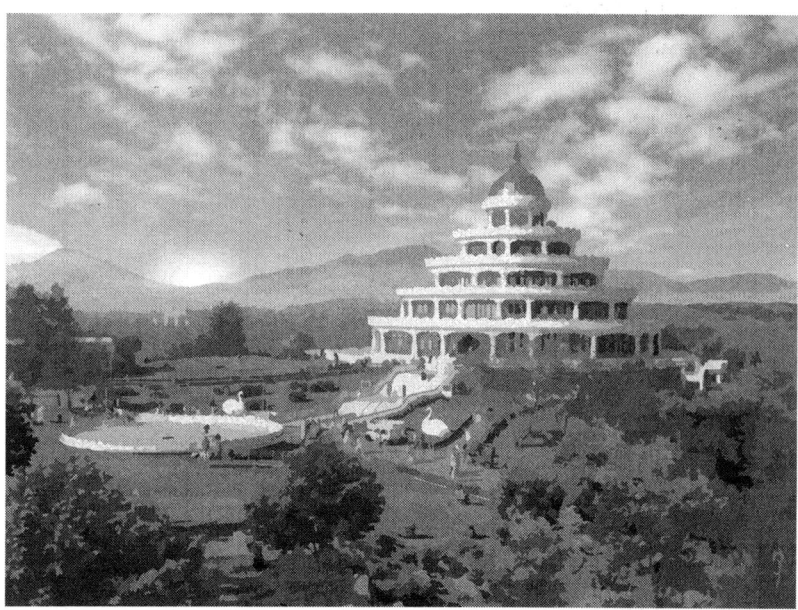

Soon he was joining the evening satsangs with Gurudev, and almost by osmosis, started meditating. He himself once wondered how and why he had suddenly started to meditate. It happened because he immersed himself each evening in the environment. Instead of sitting at home and watching TV, he started with what he enjoyed—a walk in a beautiful setting. Add in those mouthwatering pizzas, and he became an even more regular visitor to the ashram. The beautiful music in satsang, and Gurudev's inimitable style of mixing humour and mischief while He talked about the deep and profound mysteries of life became an irresistible combination for him. When he tasted meditation in this amazing setting, he wanted more. He became a meditator.

What was interesting was that it was the exact same technique he had learned decades ago that he was now diligently practising. Back then, in IIT, it was not 'cool' to meditate. It was considered a waste of time. You were labelled 'weird'. People went so far as to think you were part of some cult. Even with the best of intentions, a lot of people give up on meditation, even though they knew it was a habit that was contributing immense positivity to their lives. They preferred to belong and fit in, and give up on something truly precious than be an outlier.

Environment matters much more than you think it does.

If you want to kick an old habit, make it difficult to do and associate pain with it.

I finally beat my sugar cravings by getting rid of all the chocolates and sweet treats in my cupboard. Then even when I felt low, I knew I didn't have any chocolates at hand to binge on. It was far too much hassle to go to a shop and buy them. Chocolates were no longer an option. Instead, I would sit and do some pranayama to soothe and calm myself.

This took care of the energy conservation bit.

To make it painful for myself, if I had anything with sugar, I decided to give Rs 1000 to a cause I didn't approve of, or care about. Giving them a thousand bucks would feel horrible. Sugar stopped tasting sweet.

I have to admit that after a few months of being off sugar, I finally gave myself permission to have artisanally made dark chocolate, that too, never more than one or two pieces in a day. Out of curiosity, I tried some other sweets, platefuls of which I would have gleefully gobbled up just a year ago. I found them disgustingly, sickly sweet. My tongue had regained its innocence and I didn't like or require the humungous amounts of sweet I was previously accustomed to. In fact, I realised that I was enjoying my food even more now, because I could make out the finer differences in flavour and seasoning. The soft, subtle explosions of taste of

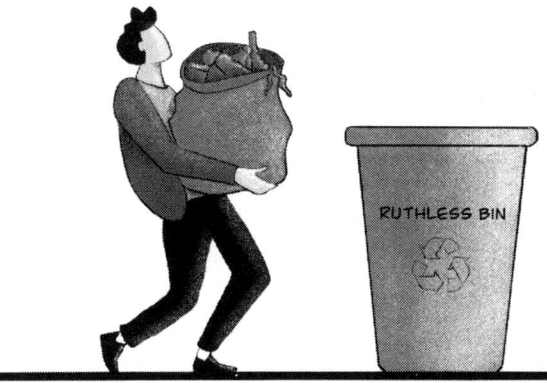

SUBTRACT STUFF FROM YOUR ENVIRONMENT - WHATEVER AND WHOEVER DON'T SERVE THE PURPOSE OF REALIZING YOUR GOALS AND DREAMS. RUTHLESSLY DELETE. YOU WILL DRAMATICALLY ADD TO THE QUALITY OF YOUR LIFE

simply cooked food were infinitely better than the relentless battering of sweet, overly spiced and salty meals. I wondered how I had eaten so much of that junk for such a long time as I pushed a plate of uneaten gulab jamun away from me.

By subtracting stuff from my environment, whatever and whoever didn't serve my purpose, I was adding to the quality of my life.

You can too.

What quality of life improvement are you seeking?

What will you subtract?

Good Night!

Dancing with Dopamine

I used to get headaches—terrible pounding, throbbing headaches. My trigger was hair. As soon as my hair would grow longer than I was used to—and I used to have really short hair—I would start to get that agonising pain in my head. It wouldn't let up until I went to a barber and got my hair trimmed. As soon as the barber was done with me, my headache would vanish.

It was really strange.

Life continued. I became an Art of Living teacher and taught meditation and the secrets of great health to scores of people. I would feel quite uncomfortable telling people that if they did meditation, they would experience far better health than they could imagine. I knew my headaches were a function of the length of my hair, and even though I had been meditating for 3-4 years, long hair resulted in horrendous pain. I started feeling like a fraud.

I had to do something about this. I decided I would grow my hair.

In a few weeks, the headaches started.

Around that time, one of the first-ever online multi-player role-playing games called Everquest had been released. It was a game almost made for me—you could play as humans, dwarves or elves … And you adventured in a fantasy world teeming with monsters—from rogue goblins and dark elves to giant ogres and even a dragon, all waiting to be slain by your heroic hand. Not only that—because it was online and multi-player, you could form a party with people from all over the world and together smash those fiends. This virtual world was exquisite, dangerous and huge. I spent many hours of many days in Norrath, the world of Everquest.

Amazingly, when I would play, there would be no headache. Over time, I noticed, even when I was not playing, the intensity of the headaches had reduced.

My hair grew, I became a well-known druid on my server in Everquest, people in real life loved my Art of Living courses, my headaches went away and life was great. It still is.

I didn't mean to keep my hair long once I had managed to grow it and not have headaches, and proved my point to myself. But too many people complimented me on my new look, and I promptly became a football of their opinions and since then have kept my hair long.

How did my headaches vanish?

I have thought about that question innumerable times and I feel I have a theory now. Of course, my regular meditation played a big part. But something else was secretly complementing my meditation. I inadvertently used my own biochemistry to my advantage, though I had no idea then that I was doing it. I feel it was dopamine that did the trick!

Rats

Dopamine is a reward hormone secreted in the brain. Every time you finish doing something, you get a squirt of it. Dopamine is the ultimate feel-good drug. There is nothing quite like it.

A bunch of rats in a lab had the dopamine centres in their brain wired to spurt the stuff each time they pressed a lever. These rats kept pressing the lever. They pressed it 800 times an hour! They didn't eat food. They didn't drink water. Their life's goal became pressing the lever to get their fix of dopamine. They just went on and on and on pressing that lever, until they collapsed from sheer exhaustion.

Another bunch of rats had the dopamine centres in their brain wired shut. Whatever they would do, there would be no dopamine. These rats became vegetables. They didn't even move to get food or water that was put near them, preferring to starve. The only time they ate food was if it was physically put into their mouths. Without the squirt of dopamine, they lost the will to eat food for their basic survival. They actually died of thirst.

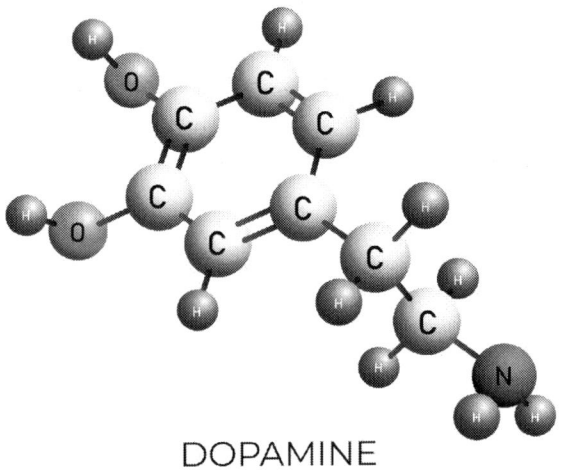

DOPAMINE

This experiment gives you a sense of the power of dopamine.[1] Almost anything you do, you do it to get that dopamine gush. Even the anticipation of an impending reward will give you a dopamine high. If you do some action,

---

[1] Of course, it's not quite as simple as that. There are a variety of chemicals and processes in the brain that will get together to create this effect, but dopamine is the key player and so we will keep it simple for this book and speak only of dopamine.

and you don't know the outcome of that action and you get a favourable result through that action, you will get an even bigger splash of the good stuff.

For example, you post a story on Instagram. A few minutes later, you check how many likes, shares and comments you have on that story. Before checking, you have no idea how many will be there. If you check and find that you have many more than you expected, you experience a thrill. Wow! People like what I posted. The wow factor! That thrill you feel is dopamine.

You are reading a brilliant book. It's late at night, and you know you should put the book away and sleep. You think, *One more page, then I will go to sleep*. Then one more, and one more and yet one more, until you fall asleep from sheer exhaustion, the book still in your hands. Sounds quite like those rats we talked about earlier, doesn't it? This is dopamine at work. The sheer delight of getting to know what happens next keeps you awake way past your bedtime.

You are idly scrolling through Facebook or Instagram. You think, let me check out one more post, read one more story and then I will sit and work on that presentation. And suddenly it's 2 a.m. Blame it on dopamine.

Dopamine can make you do stuff that you would usually not think of doing if you were thinking rationally. And yet, without dopamine, you are zombified. You will not even want to get out of bed.

Everquest

Everquest was a gorgeously designed game. Each encounter was almost a perfect challenge throughout the game. If your foes had their names in green, they were easy to vanquish, the ones with blue names were tough if you were alone, though easy to plough through if you were playing with even one more person. The monsters who had white names were touch and go, and the ones who were red would almost certainly beat you.

When adventuring solo, you would stick to greens, blues and the occasional white if you were feeling really brave. But in groups you could, with careful coordination, take on the reds. I would decide to play for an hour to escape the headache and end up playing four hours straight. The dopamine rush was incredible. So incredible that my head would even forget to ache because of my growing hair!

I have always led a full life replete with exciting challenges. While dealing with headaches and playing Everquest, I was involved in organising and teaching Art of Living courses. I was busy creating vegetarian delicacies for my then non-vegetarian family in an effort to sway them towards a cleaner, greener, healthier lifestyle. I was practising and prepping for a piano performance. There were many things in life other than Everquest that would give me my dopamine rush. I had the good sense to get involved in life far more than I was involved in the game.

A few of my friends who used to play with me were not as lucky as I was.

They didn't have much going in their lives and the world of Everquest sucked them into a vortex of dopamine. They would play the whole day and most of the night. They hardly slept. They ate junk, drank alcohol and totally abused themselves. While others in our friend circle were getting jobs and starting businesses, these guys were getting wasted. They never realised the harm they were doing to themselves while they gleefully battled yet another monstrosity in Norrath.

Rats again.

Action Addiction

While it may not get as extreme as it did for a few of those unlucky people I knew, you may get caught up in what I call action addiction. Have you had days when you were busy throughout the day, rushing from one task to another, to another, to yet another? You felt drained at the end of that hectic workday. But pause and reflect for a bit about what you actually managed to accomplish that day, and you will find that all those frenetic actions actually added up to almost nothing.

I did so much work, yet I did nothing.

People get caught up in the small, mundane, pointless activities of life. Checking emails and promptly answering them, keeping a tab on WhatsApp, Slack, Telegraph, Elyments and other messenger apps, checking LinkedIn, Twitter, Facebook, Instagram and other social media, reading the news, flipping channels and watching TV, attending meetings, being constantly watchful about any of those notification alerts that pop up, writing out reports, going for marriages ... the list of things to do is endless. You finish one, three more pop up. You get busier and busier doing almost nothing that adds up to your big dream. If this is you, know that you too are a victim of dopamine. Those little sprays you get each time you get something done, and off your infinite to-do list, end up making you into a hardcore addict.

Dopamine will wrench you away from the bigger goals of your life by drugging you into the complacency of busyness.

Think about all you dream about—you wanted to start that side business, learn to play the guitar, cook something exotic, become fitter, read those books, spend more time with the people you love, go for a vacation and really unwind ... all these get swept away into the fire of dopamine. You constantly console yourself that you will start tomorrow, or after a week, or next year while tapping away on your phone, replying to yet another WhatsApp message.

Unfortunately, it doesn't end here. Like any addiction, as it becomes a habit for you to go about your day in a frenzy of activity, you will get accustomed to the high levels of dopamine coursing through your blood. As time goes by, you will require even more sprays of dopamine to give you that high you have become helplessly hooked on to. This translates into even more pointless frenzied activity. You are not too far from those rats pressing a lever. The only difference is that you are pressing hundreds of little levers you have created for yourself—not just one. In truth, there is not much to distinguish between you and my friends from long ago who got wasted playing Everquest.

Dopamine Detox

Inconsequential small things are piling up and just have to get done. You feel rushed and tired and even though you are constantly on the move, you feel like you are on a merry-go-round—going round and round, faster and faster and are still in the same old place. If days, weeks and months are just flying by and you are nowhere closer to where you want to be in life, it is highly probable that you are a victim of action addiction.

The first step is to accept that you are indeed addicted. Once acceptance dawns, there is hope for intelligent action. In this case though, the intelligent action is inaction. Start with just a day of being offline. No phone, no internet, no gadget. You are welcome to read a book, go for a walk, exercise ... do anything other than what you are accustomed to doing.

For a full day. 24 hours.

You may use the time to plan out stuff in life—what you are going to do, when, for how long, with whom. Even to make these notes, do not use gadgets. Use pen and paper.

Once the 24 hours are up, go back to your gadgets for a week or so. Then once more, detach for a day. Continue like this for 3-4 weeks. In the second month, do the gadget detox for 2-5 days. A perfect opportunity to do an Art of Living advanced meditation programme. Or go off for a vacation for a few days, to a place where there is little to no internet access.

As your dopamine levels fall and you are no longer accustomed to those crazy highs, you will see that your action addiction is under control. You will find that you don't need to do quite so many pointless things in a day to get your dopamine rush. If you feel like you are slipping out of control again, a digital detox day will fix you. Five days offline, twice or thrice a year, will reset your dopamine cravings, so you are not addicted anymore and can think straight and take part in smart action.

Leveraging Dopamine

Remember that dopamine is chiefly secreted by three triggers:
1. You anticipate a reward
2. You get something done
3. You perform an action and there is a probability that the result of that action is in your favour. The higher the odds against you, the more satisfying the dopamine kick if it does swing in your favour.

And remember that like any other addictive substance, over time you will need more and more of it to get the high you are used to.

Put all this together and it becomes simple and obvious about how to use the awesome power of dopamine to your advantage.

If you did the Pizza of Life process then you should be having a fairly clear idea about where you want to be in life. Your identity and vision of how your life would be could be considered as a long-term project. Let's say one of the things you want to be is a well-known author.

Being an author means you need to write at least one book. And let's define well-known as having at least 15,000 copies of the book sold.

Your project now has two parts to it—one part is about figuring out what book you want to write and the second is about how you are going to ensure it gets sold once you do finish writing it.

Each part can be broken down into tasks. Each task is chunked into actions.

For example, for the book writing, a broad overview of the tasks could be:
- Deciding the topic, assuming you have decided to write a non-fiction book
- Researching and making notes about the topic
- Creating a skeletal outline of the book
- Deciding what topics will definitely be in the book, or what may be in the final book and what will not be part of the book
- Going back and doing even more research with all this in mind
- Starting to jot down ideas as they come, so they can be developed later as you continue to research
- Writing out a chapter or two you feel are easy for you to write

- Sending those out to a few friends who can give you feedback and with whom you can discuss the direction the book is going to take
- Continuing to write and develop chapters
- Deciding about illustrations—whether your book will have them or not
- Finding someone to do illustrations and the book cover
- Geting into the research, writing, getting feedback, rewriting if required and going back to research loop
- Seeing how everything is coming together once your first draft is done—getting into ruthless edit mode and chucking whatever doesn't contribute to the aim of the book
- Writing or rewriting whatever is required
- Getting the final manuscript ready to send to editors—who may suggest improvements to language and grammar
- Doing the back and forth with editors to create a polished final version
- Having my entire book read out to me a few times so I know how it will sound in the head of the person who is going to read it, and while this reading is going on, I will continue to edit to make it sound even better
- Approving, disapproving or tweaking illustrations and the book cover
- Sending off the book for printing
- Praying that people will love it

If you have never published a book before, there is an entire exercise of meeting various publishers and pitching your book in the hope that they will accept it, and agree to publish it. Some authors may choose to go the self-publishing route, and will require to do research on that. This phase requires a lot of exploration in its own right at least the first few times.

Now calendarise these tasks, giving yourself a sort of schedule about when what needs to get done. Give yourself plenty of flexibility on this—it's just broad strokes so you know approximately how long it's going to take, and more or less when you will do what. You could modify this schedule as you get moving, and make it tighter once you know how good you are at pacing your work.

Boil all this down to what actions you will take this month, this week and finally, what you will do today. Notice that now you have a list of actions that need to be done on an everyday basis that will actually contribute towards your greater goal of being an author.

Perform those actions consistently each day, every day, until they become a habit.

5½ Minutes

Don't underestimate the power of doing small things consistently over an appreciable period of time. I present a bit of math to make my point.

$1^{365} = 1$

1 raised to 365 – meaning 1 x 1 x 1 x 1 ... 365 times is just 1.

But check this out:

$1.01^{365} = 37.8$

And $0.99^{365} = 0.03$

What does this mean?

If you continue to do whatever it is that you are doing, after a year you will be more or less where you are now. But add just 1% of extra effort each day and you will have approximately thirty-eight times more than what you have now when the year is over.

Think of what this means. If you have a normal nine-hour working day, this means you are working approximately 540 minutes each day. 1% of 540 minutes is 5½ minutes. If you can spend 5½ minutes each day doing some small action that will take you towards improving your scores on the Pizza of Life, at the end of the year you will have 38 times more than what you started with.

It can go quite wrong as well. Slip up just 1% doing whatever you are doing each day, and by the end of the year you will be approximately 1,200 times worse off than you would be if you had been putting in that 1% daily.

If you consistently do small things which are geared towards you becoming that person you always wanted to be, know that in time this will be inevitable. Time is key here.

When I am learning a new piece of music on the piano, it doesn't come together in a day or two or three. First, I will learn the music for each hand separately. When I am confident that I can play both hands separately, I will gingerly put them together—really slowly. Once I have the rhythm of how the notes work when both hands are playing together, I will bring in the pedal and increase speed over a few days of practice. When I have the speed and am confident of the way I am playing, I will put in expression—being louder, softer, slower and faster at different places so the music really comes alive.

Many times I don't notice the small incremental improvements in my playing from one day to the next. I keep feeling I am making the same mistakes again and again. Sometimes a particularly aggravating part could take days to get just right. But when it does come together, it always feels that it suddenly happened, and sounds amazing that day.

Somewhere I know that it's sounding fantastic because of all those hours of practice that went into it for weeks or months. But when that magic finally transpires, you think it happened in that moment.

While planning out this part of the book, I actually allowed myself to practice a piece of music for just 5½ minutes each day. I was amazed that within a month of doing this, I knew it and was playing it really well! This was much, much better than I had dared to hope.

That's when I knew 5½ minutes a day can be pure magic.

Take the top three priorities in your Pizza of Life. Give them each 5½ minutes a day.

Thank me after a year!

As far as the brain is concerned, you are getting things done in those 5½ minutes. It will reward you with those dopamine squirts and make you feel fantastic. It's an amazing loop to get into—get some meaningful stuff done and enjoy the dopamine kick that spurs you on to getting even more meaningful stuff done. Rinse and repeat.

And by the way, you don't have to stop after 5½ minutes each day ... That's just how you start.

This is the way dopamine was supposed to work for you. Give you a high that spurs you along as each little thing gets done, and falls into place. Word by word, line by line, chapter by chapter, soon you will have written a book. You will have become an author.

Congratulations! You have conquered action addiction. Or have you?

Mistake

Most people make a big mistake in this process. They postpone their celebration to the very end—only when that big project is completed. They think, *When the book is complete, I will go on a vacation.* This strategy conveys to the brain that the small actions that you do towards that big goal are unworthy of celebration.

If there is no reward as each chapter is completed, for example, you will find it more and more difficult to write. That big reward at the end is too far away, too unreachable. And no reward after finishing a chapter means you are telling the brain it's no big deal. You will hardly get any dopamine then. Without dopamine, you quickly lose interest, and your brain will literally force you into some pointless activity or the other so that you can get your dopamine fix. Fall into this trap and you can forget about the book and any other dream you might have. You end up as prey of your own biochemistry.

Instead, celebrate the small wins—a big piece of chocolate whenever a chapter is completed or a pizza and movie night with friends when you finish writing a particularly difficult piece or a humungous glass of mango milkshake or an extra hour of video games when you are happy with everything you accomplished that day. Whatever reward makes sense to you is fine.

This reward reinforces the habit for your brain which will then happily give you your dose of dopamine. And sooner than you can imagine, you will be what you have been wanting to be.

Rewards

Let's talk about video games again. A well-designed game will reward you when you complete a particular task. If you are a wizard, you will get a new spell or an upgraded version of something you already have—the spark becomes a fireball. So you can be even more formidable in battle as you continue to tackle the more dangerous critters in the game. After completing a level, would it make sense to reward the wizard with a sword he cannot use? Of course not! The reward needs to grant a significant advantage to the character as he continues his quest, or it is no reward at all.

But check out how people tend to reward themselves in real life.

I want to be fit. I lost a kilo through exercise. Reward? A BIG piece of chocolate cake! This is like giving a sword to a wizard instead of a wand. This is completely pointless and counterproductive to the ultimate goal of being fit.

Instead, how about this? I lost a kilo through exercise. Reward? A new pair of gym shoes to train in.

As you celebrate your small victories, let the celebrations be in sync with your dream. Let your rewards augment you towards your ultimate goal and not take you away from it.

Learn to dance with dopamine without giving in to its mesmeric charms and you will be able to leverage its astounding power to your advantage.

What actions will you perform today? Even if they are for just 5½ minutes …

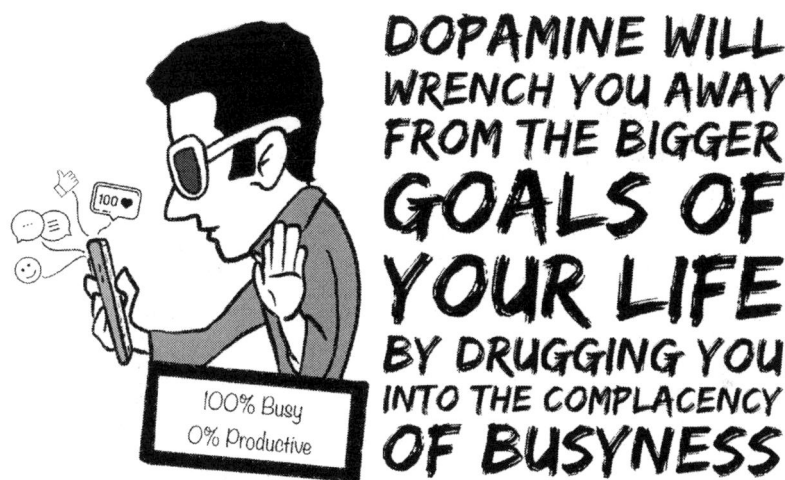

Will you be closer to your dream tonight than you were in the morning?

How will you celebrate?

Good Night!

Allies and Power-ups

My team and I were in charge of organising a public event, a satsang for Gurudev Sri Sri Ravi Shankar in Mumbai. We had booked a huge open-air venue so we could accommodate the tens of thousands of people who would come to meet Him. The city of Mumbai was plastered with posters and we even had a few hoardings. We worked as hard as we possibly could—letting everyone know about the event, inviting them and assuring them that it would be an evening to remember.

Finally, the day of the event dawned. We were all stretched to the limit—caught up in the last-minute rush of getting things in place for a perfect event. It was a balmy summer evening. A cool breeze blew. The stage was elegantly decorated. The sound system was perfectly set up. The musicians had started singing. Gurudev's car pulled up and He floated regally onto the stage …

Everything was picture perfect.

There was just one thing missing.

Given the size of the setting, it felt as if there was hardly anyone in the audience.

The venue looked stark. Almost empty. Where there should have been over a hundred thousand people, there were not even twenty thousand.

Gurudev didn't bat an eyelid. He conducted the satsang as if the grounds were packed. He stayed for the entire two-hour duration of the programme. He spoke about the profound wisdom of Indian spirituality in His characteristic light, humourous way. Then He led everyone into deep, deep transcendental states of meditation. Everyone there was transported to some alternate reality.

Except me.

I knew we had messed up. I was feeling terrible about letting Gurudev down and utterly embarrassed about the poor turnout. I was definitely not looking forward to the inevitable admonishment I was going to get pretty soon.

All too soon, the satsang was over, and as He was stepping off the stage, He beckoned me and asked me to join him in the car.

I had been dreading this moment. With great trepidation, I got into the car with Him. He didn't reprimand me in any way. Instead, He asked how the satsang had gone. I said it had been surreal and magical.

There was a long pause.

Then He looked at me straight in the eyes and said, 'Why were there so few people? What went wrong?'

I knew what had gone wrong. My ego had made me choose to work with just a few people I was comfortable with, thinking we would manage to pull off the event. I had not reached out for support and involved as many people as I could from the Art of Living organisation in Mumbai.

I said to Him simply, 'Gurudev, I didn't involve everyone. I thought we could do this by ourselves.'

He held my gaze, then gently smiled and said, 'Good. You have learned something from this. When would you like to organise the next big event?'

He looked at His calendar and gave me a date around three months later. And that was it.

This time around, I ensured we had reached out to absolutely everyone. We had a huge team, and though there were the inevitable clashes, everyone managed to work together mostly coherently. The feeling and energy of a really big team working towards a mutual goal was amazing.

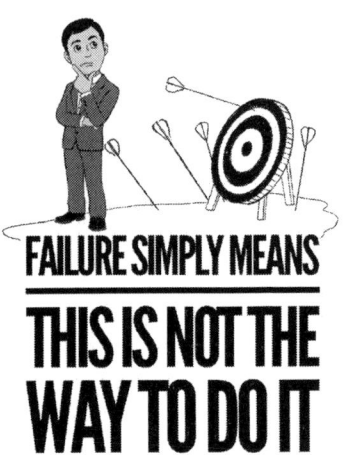

FAILURE SIMPLY MEANS THIS IS NOT THE WAY TO DO IT

Those three months whooshed past and all too soon the day of the event was upon us.

That evening, almost an hour before we were ready to start, the grounds were full. There must have been more than 150,000 people. As Gurudev walked on to the stage that evening, He caught my eye and smiled. It was a gorgeous event, an outstanding success.

Later, as I was mulling over all that had happened, I began to realise that I couldn't consider the first event as a failure. It had actually been a carefully crafted opportunity for me to learn. Gurudev had graciously allowed me to fail, so I could understand that I need to keep my ego aside and work with anyone, not just people I am comfortable with.

Here is a parenting tip if there ever was one. As children grow older, they need to become all right with failing. Too many parents overprotect their children, shielding them from failure. There has to be a point when parents need to let go. They need to let their children fail, if required, so they could learn from that experience. Sometimes children might learn a valuable life lesson only through a fiasco. Great parenting is knowing when to allow the child to fall, yet be ready to catch them as they fall!

This Is Not the Way to Do It

Through my life, I have had some spectacular failures. Each time I have learned something. And if I have learned something truly valuable, can I honestly call the experience a failure?

For me, failure has become an opportunity to learn, to grow.

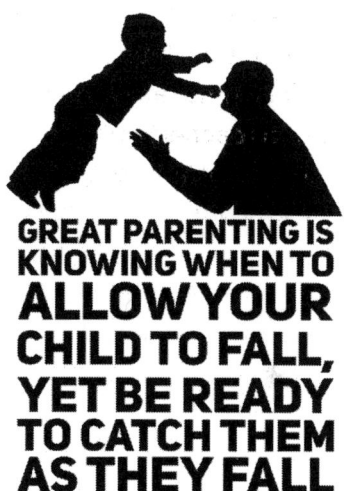

GREAT PARENTING IS KNOWING WHEN TO ALLOW YOUR CHILD TO FALL, YET BE READY TO CATCH THEM AS THEY FALL

When you refuse to learn from a failure or a mistake, you get into trouble. Then you have truly failed. It is quite incredible how so many people refuse to learn from mistakes—their own, or other people's—doing the same thing over and over again, expecting different results every time. Isn't this insanity?

Failure simply means what you are doing is not the way to do a certain thing.

If you screwed up, do it some other way. Keep finding new ways until you manage to figure out how to do a certain thing, or that what you were attempting to do is simply not possible. That could be a learning as well.

Unfortunately, most people have made failure out to be 'bad'. You are made to feel ashamed that you failed. The emotional charge that is created by failure is hugely magnified by the people around us. Most people end up fearing failure.

This is a costly mistake.

I feel this attitude towards failure is the reason why the vast majority of the population the world over is stuck in middle-class mediocrity. People are so scared that they might fail that they don't want to take risks. Most don't even begin on their dreams, and settle for a safe humdrum existence.

They don't realise that the risk of failure is intrinsically built into anything big and truly worth achieving. Only a brave person who is all right to fail can play big. Note that they don't start expecting to fail. They are just reconciled to the fact that failure is possible.

The others, they watch and wonder how resounding success keeps eluding them, even though they are 'good, hardworking, honest' people …

Video Games

Ever played a video game?

My favourite type of game to play is an RPG—a role playing game. You fire the game up and are thrust into a fantastic alternate reality—it could be deep space or it could be some medieval fantasy realm. You have some goals to accomplish, and little to no idea about how you are going to do it.

You might have woken up from some cryogenic slumber on an abandoned spaceship. You cannot remember how you got there, or even who you are, and need to find out what happened and how to get back home. Or you start off as a lowly farmer in some small village who suddenly discovers that he can create fireballs and lightning while defending his flock of sheep from a pack of hungry wolves. The farmer turns out to be the one the Gods were looking for to deliver the universe from an evil dark force threatening to snuff out all beings of light, and from your humble beginnings you embark on a fabulous adventure to save the world … and your sheep!

There are other types of more 'casual' games—the 'Match 3' where you need to match three or more of the same type of icons to have them pop away, or the space invaders type, where you fight with all sorts of alien ships wanting to destroy you and they come at you faster and faster as the game progresses.

Then there are the city building games, where you design a city and provide education, jobs, food, etc. for your virtual population and build roads that minimize traffic jams.

Check out the Google Play Store or the Apple App Store for a plethora of games you could play …

There is one thing that is common through any game you play.

All video games are designed to make you fail.

Some of them like Flappy Bird are set up in such a way that in the first few seconds of playing you know you will lose. You start the game knowing you will lose, the point being to see how far you can go before inevitable defeat. Flappy Bird is one of the most frustratingly difficult games I have ever played and that's why I enjoyed it.

Others are a little more forgiving—Sky Force, for example, is a shooting game that makes you lose, unless you get it just right. It is a challenge to clear all the levels with the highest possible scores.

Still others are more sympathetic, and draw you into their worlds with just the right amount of tension thrown in … though any really good game would intrinsically have a huge risk of failure before getting to the final goal expertly woven into it.

Almost all video games have a few aspects in common—they have something called power-ups—a magic potion, or an enchanted diamond, or a super charged fuel tank or a few seconds of hyper fire power that either helps recover the hero from almost fatal damage or helps him fight an enemy clearly bigger, meaner and more powerful than he could ever hope to be. These power-ups help to tide over the really tough sections of the game. By design, they are rare to find, and so must be saved for emergencies.

Then there are allies—your friends who help you in your quest. They augment your skills and make your in-game life much easier. Along with your hero, they too need nurturing, so that they grow in power, and become true assets in helping your hero move successfully to their ultimate goal.

The story and characters in the story, the balance of difficulty, the right amount of risk of failure, the rarity and potency of the power-ups and the supplementation of your skills by your allies all come together to create a wondrous memorable gaming experience.

World of Warcraft, an iconic massively multiplayer role-playing game has over 5 million players playing since it was launched in November 2004. The total number of hours that we, as humans, have spent playing it actually exceeds the number of hours we, as a species, have been on planet Earth!

When you finish a well-crafted game, there is a sense of exhilaration. You beat the huge dragon. You destroyed the evil cyborg. You annihilated the dark lord. You designed an exquisite garden. You built a magnificent empire.

You fought. You tried again and again. You failed. You didn't give up. You strategised. You designed. You created. You won.

Now, just think about this—would you feel even a fraction of that high if the game was too simple? If you knew as you started the game that you were going to beat it easily, there would almost be no point playing it. Realise that the feeling you feel when you emerge a winner from a well-designed game is created because there was that risk of failure forever looming over your head. Remove that, and the game fails to engage you.

There are millions and millions of people who play games every day. And all these millions of people know this.

But, unfortunately, these millions of people have not made the connection of playing games to their own lives.

Gamifying Life

The Brahmasutras say, *'Lokavattu leela kaivalyam.'* The whole world is nothing but a game. Did our ancient Rishis play video games too?! ☺

At any given point of time, we have challenges and goals.

The promotion you are working for. The business you have always wanted to start. The entrance exam you want to pass. The relationship with someone special you are intent upon creating. The financial freedom you wish you had. The great health you want to enjoy. The book you want to write. The film you want to make …

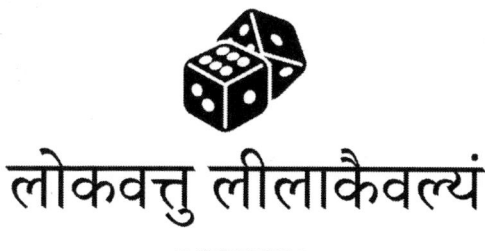

These are the dragons that need slaying, the cities that need building.

We have people in our lives who help us as we strive to get to our goal—our allies. We depend on these people. They give us strength. They make us feel good. They are there with us when things get tough. These are the relationships that need to be nurtured and cultivated. A great hero is only as powerful as his allies are.

It's worth pausing and thinking about all those who truly matter to you in your life.

Are you making time for them? Relationships need care and attention to blossom.

All too often, we spend too much of our time with people who don't contribute significantly to our lives. Many times, they may even be parasites—the ones who take you for granted or insult or provoke you and make you feel terrible about yourself.

One of the biggest rules of my life is simple— I spend maximum time with people who make me feel good and minimise the time with people who don't. I make time for my allies. I show them I care, and that they are special to me. I don't just think about this. I do it.

It was not always like this. At one time, I used to spend far too much of myself on people who simply didn't care for me as much as I cared for them. I did all the heavy lifting in the relationship. This meant that I didn't have as much time for the people who truly mattered, and I ended up taking my allies for granted. I made the people who made me feel great feel unwanted. Thankfully, these people were true allies and stayed on while I sorted things out in my life.

I slowly drifted out of toxic relationships. I freed myself up for my allies, becoming an ally for them in their lives. I recognised that just as I was the hero of my life, they were the heroes of theirs and needed a great ally too.

On a side note, this doesn't mean that I don't work with people I may not get along with too well. That's a different story altogether. When it's inevitable that I need to work with someone, however obnoxious they are, so that a greater good can be manifested, I do it with good grace.

At the beginning of each year, when people are making their new year's resolutions, I make my list of people I am grateful for. People whom I love to be with. People who give me courage and strength. People who care. People who matter. People who I can be completely honest with. People who make me laugh and feel free. Through the year, I ensure that I spend quality time with all these wonderful people I have been blessed with in my life. My life and theirs is so much better because of this.

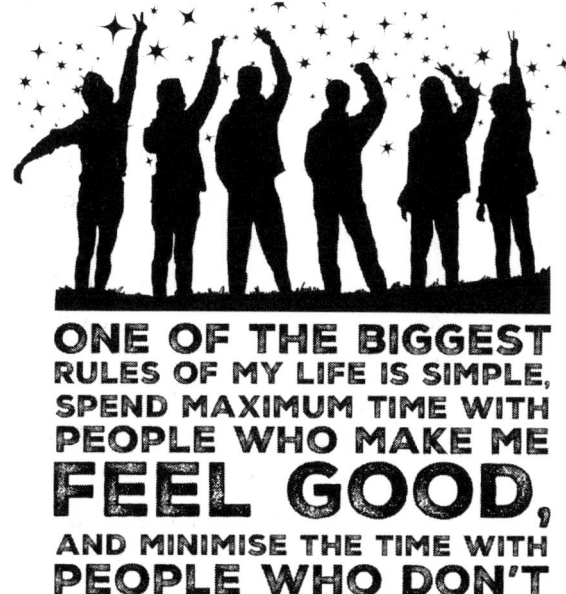

ONE OF THE BIGGEST RULES OF MY LIFE IS SIMPLE, SPEND MAXIMUM TIME WITH PEOPLE WHO MAKE ME FEEL GOOD, AND MINIMISE THE TIME WITH PEOPLE WHO DON'T

It would be a great idea for you to write out the names of at least five people who matter to you—whom you know you can depend on and who know that they can depend on you.

My allies
1.
2.
3.
4.
5.

Feel free to add to this list. A huge list will enrich your life beyond anything you can imagine. Once you have the names jotted down, make a habit of developing these relationships.

Raindrops on Roses and Whiskers on Kittens ...

Along with great allies we need strong power-ups.

There are going to be times in life when everything feels unfair. When things are difficult. When you hit rock bottom. When there doesn't seem to be any glimmer of hope or light.

When you are feeling down and out, you will not have the energy to even think about things that make you feel better. Having an inventory of power-ups ready could become a superb asset to pull you through tough times.

What makes you feel resourced? On your worst day, what could still bring a smile to your lips? Which actions? What memories? Make a list. Keep it safe and handy. Keep adding to your list.

Most people, when they are feeling low, will listen to sad songs. This vibes with their mood, but will only create even more gloom within them, locking them up in their misery for that much longer. Don't do this. Do what Julie Andrews does in the movie *The Sound of Music* instead. She sings the lovely song, 'These are a few of my favourite things' when the children in her care are upset and afraid. You too play happy songs instead, and you will quickly realise the potency of a great power-up.

Do this one thing for sure. Create a playlist of uplifting, upbeat music; songs you enjoy singing or humming along with the track; songs that are about happiness, sunshine, flowers, beauty, peace and love. Have at least twenty songs in that playlist. The next time you are feeling down and out, just hit the play button on this playlist. For the first few minutes, you will hate listening to all that joy when you are feeling so miserable about whatever is going on with you. Then memories will start kicking in, and suddenly that dark mood will lift as you will not be able to help but be carried along by the music. The cobwebs will clear, and you will begin to feel better much faster than you could have imagined. Sound affects space, and we all are made up of 98% space.

Here is a snippet from my list of power-ups in no particular order to get you started.

1. Memories of Arosa in Switzerland with Gurudev
2. Rafting on the Ganga
3. Reading P.G. Wodehouse
4. Listening to Mozart, Chopin, Beethoven, Liszt and Schubert
5. A playlist of my happy songs
6. Harshal singing
7. Baked pumpkin with tahini
8. A neat, clean room and desk
9. The smell of night jasmine
10. Mangoes
11. More mangoes
12. Massages
13. Long walks
14. Playing with dogs and cats
15. Dark chocolate
16. Beaches
17. Craniosacral Therapy
18. Even more mangoes
19. Sunsets
20. Bach Flower Essences
21. Waterfalls
22. Green smoothies made by Dinesh
23. Flying business class
24. Pedicures

25. Full moon nights
26. Monsoon in the Sahyadris
27. Watching funny movies and musicals
28. Candles
29. The Art of Living ashrams in Bangalore, Rishikesh and Germany
30. Going shopping
31. I did mention mangoes, didn't I?! ☺

An inventory of heavy-duty power-ups and rock-solid allies will give you the confidence to take calculated risks. You will know that you have a support system in place, just in case you fail, and you will not be afraid to create a stunning reality for yourself.

Just remember—God is the greatest game designer ever. Everything has been put perfectly in place for a grand adventure.

Now reach for the stars!

Good Night!

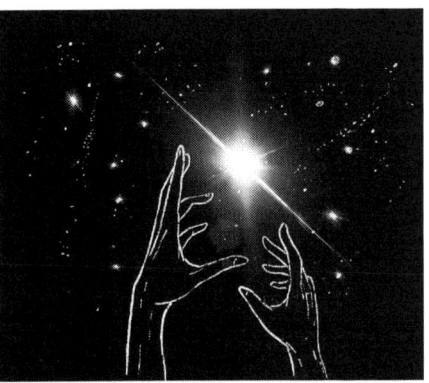

GOD IS THE GREATEST GAME DESIGNER EVER. EVERYTHING HAS BEEN PUT PERFECTLY IN PLACE FOR A GRAND ADVENTURE. NOW REACH FOR THE STARS

Karma and Destiny

In a nutshell, Karma simply means that for any action, even an inaction, there will be consequences. This is what keeps things fair and sane. And the world chugs along merrily.

If this was not the case, when the husband asks his wife, 'Honey, what are we having for dinner?', she will have to say, 'No idea, darling. I put rice in the cooker; God knows what we will get.'

If you put rice in the cooker, you will get cooked rice, burnt rice or undercooked rice for dinner. You will not get pizza. At least not from the cooker. This is Karma.

Some Karma is realised quickly. Other Karma takes time. Plant coriander seeds and you get leaves for a tasty chutney within 2 weeks or so. Plant a mango tree and you have to wait 5 years or more to begin to enjoy all that summery goodness.

Karma also means impression. Do you have the habit of having coffee every morning? Having coffee every morning, day after day, for years on end, will kind of make a figurative groove in your consciousness. You will have developed coffee Karma.

Some actions have to be done consistently over time to see results—lifting a few weights in the gym for three days will not give you huge biceps. You will need to work out consistently, and only in time will you see the difference.

Similarly, if you have been doing bodybuilding for a prolonged period of time and created a fantastic physique for yourself, you will not suddenly deflate if you don't exercise for a month.

This is why it's so difficult to suddenly give up on that coffee.

However, no karmic effect is indefinite. In time, the consequence of any action will dissipate. Even a huge boulder thrown into a lake cannot create waves and ripples forever. In time, all disturbance will subside.

Your actions create consequences not just for you but for many around you. A doctor saving the life of a man will affect that man's entire family, his business and all who come in contact with him. Just as your actions affect many people around you, others' actions can affect you too. The Coronavirus pandemic of 2020 is the perfect example of this. A few people's carelessness and indifference in one corner of the world created dire consequences for almost everyone on our planet.

The threads of Karma are deeply intertwined and get supremely complicated exponentially. We are all bound by Karma.

If you give this a thought, you will realise how Karma will automatically give rise to the concept of reincarnation. If you do something in this lifetime and happen to die before facing the consequence of that action, then it's carried forward to your next birth. That's what keeps things just.

People bemoan their destiny. When you begin to understand just a little about Karma, you recognise what's happening in your life is not stuff ordained by some higher power, but by you yourself! You have created your own destiny through your Karma. The Higher Power is just there to make sure you cannot escape your Karma.

Think of rice pudding. Boil rice in milk, add sugar and you get some yummy kheer, as it's called in India. At this point, you have many options—you could add more milk to liquify the consistency and lessen the sweetness. You could add more sugar. You could add vanilla essence for a European flavour or saffron for a more Indian taste. You could add dry fruits. I could go on and on, but you get the point.

What you cannot do, however, is get the original rice back. Once the rice is boiled, there is no way you are going to get the raw rice back again.

In much the same way, there are consequences of some of our actions that we simply have to face. Nature in her wisdom created a loophole, though. Exactly the way we could modify the kheer through our current actions, we can modify the consequences of our past actions as well.

Say, because of some terrible stuff you did, a stone will fall on your head.

This is fixed. The stone will fall. There is no way to escape it.

However, if you have been a nice person—helping people, doing meditation, making a positive difference to yourself and those around you, recommending this book to others, etc., the stone that falls could be just a tiny pebble—you may not even notice it. And if you have been nasty? Well then, the stone could turn out to be a rock, possibly hurrying you into your next birth, with at least this bit of karma neutralised.

Because you did something really nice, you may have the destiny of winning a lottery ticket. This will not change. You will win that prize. How much, though, is again going to depend on your recent actions—if you have been a good person, you may win in lakhs and crores. If not, you may win a hundred rupees.

Your actions right now will affect the fructification of your destiny. Nothing is ever fatalistic. Everything is always fluid.

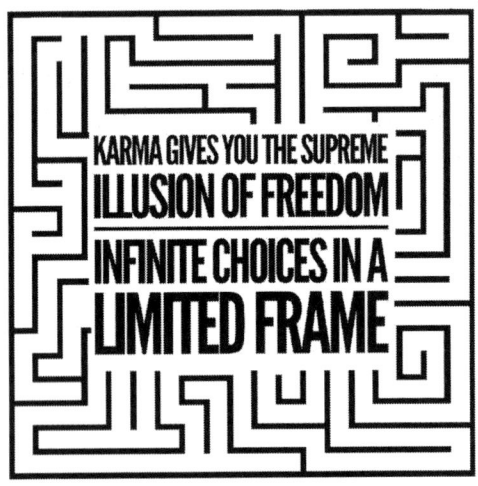

Think of being inside a circle. There are an infinite number of points inside that circle, which means at any given moment, there are an infinite number of actions available to you. There is an even bigger infinity (don't ask) of points outside that circle. This signifies that there are myriad actions that are simply not available to you at a given moment in time. For example, if you are in Bangalore, physically disappearing and suddenly appearing in London is simply not possible.

This is how Karma will bind and entwine you. It gives you infinite freedom in a limited frame, the supreme illusion of freedom.

Knowing this, think of the best possible illusion of reality you would like to create for yourself. Your actions right now will take you towards the fructification of your dream within the grand dream. You anyway have to act. Choosing not to act is an action as well, and that will create its own consequences. You might as well act and move towards creating that nicer illusion for yourself, rather than getting stuck in the illusion that you are in right now. Because until you are enlightened, all these illusions feel really real.

Enlightenment? What's that?

For an Enlightened Master, there is no circle. No Karma touches him. Though He will pretend there is, and it does. He willingly steps into the illusion so He can lead us out of it.

Good Night!

(Just in case all this is true, be nice and act—those stars await you!)

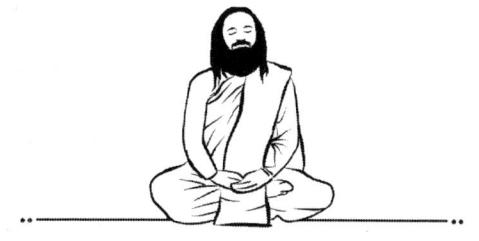

NO KARMA CAN TOUCH AN ENLIGHTENED MASTER. THOUGH HE WILL PRETEND THAT IT DOES. HE WILLINGLY STEPS INTO ILLUSION SO HE CAN LEAD US OUT OF IT.

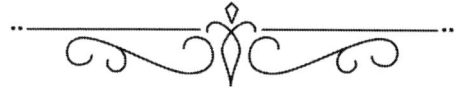

APPENDIX

Three Magic Plants for the Bedroom

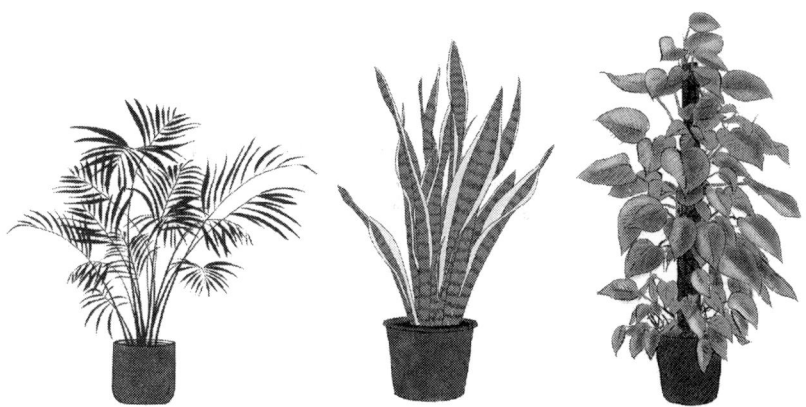

Three plants are excellent for the bedroom. All three are cheap to buy, look pretty, brighten up the space and are easy to take care of. Most importantly, they give out oxygen at night. Along with a good air purifier that rids the air of allergens, pollen, mould etc., these three plants can suffuse your space with oxygen, creating a brilliant sleeping environment.

For all three, apart from the easy-care instructions below, there is one critical thing that must be done at least twice a week. Remember to wipe down their leaves with a clean wet cloth. We want these plants to produce oxygen for us, and that's not going to happen if the leaves are covered with dust which clog their pores.

The first and easiest to maintain is *Sansevieria Trifasciata*, popularly called the snake plant, mother-in-law's tongue or Saint George's sword. It has beautiful long, stiff, dark green vertical leaves that have striking light green bands. It may sprout pretty little white flowers after a few years.

This plant can absorb toxic gases that may be present in the air in your bedroom. It doesn't need frequent watering and grows quite fast, making it a superb plant to start with if you are a beginner to indoor gardening. It is, however, toxic for dogs and cats, so if you have pets, keep this plant out of their reach.

The soil in the pot should be more or less dry and able to drain well, so water it just once or twice a month. Constant watering will rot the roots and kill it. It loves sunlight but is quite happy indoors and doesn't mind low light conditions. I have a few which I keep rotating. A few weeks in my bedroom, and then the next few weeks outside, on the terrace. Don't expose this plant to too many hours of direct sunlight. It doesn't quite like that.

The second, just as easy to maintain, is *Epipremnum Aureum*, popularly called the money plant. It is supposed to bring wealth to the home it is grown in, but urban legend says that it should be stolen from some place for that to happen.

This versatile plant requires well-draining soil and can grow up to a height of 12 feet if well cared for. Touch the top soil of the pot and only if it feels dry, water the plant—never more than once a week. You will know if you have not given it enough water when cracks appear on the surface of the soil. When this plant has been utterly neglected, it feels sorry for itself and can become droopy, its usual shiny emerald green leaves becoming a sick yellow. It is a hardy plant though, and will soon bounce back to vibrant green health if you give it the little bit of attention that it wants.

Money plants love partially shady areas and so grow quite well indoors where they can get some indirect sunlight. They grow equally well in a garden too. Some people like to grow money plants in just water. That works great as well—change the water once every week and your money plant will be thrilled.

The third plant is *Chrysalidocarpus Lutescens*, popularly called the areca palm. It is a big beautiful plant that brightens up the interiors with its bold green feathery arching fronds.

The key to maintaining a healthy areca palm is bright, indirect sunlight. Give them this and they can be quite forgiving of everything else. Like the snake plant, I rotate my areca palms every few weeks from the terrace to the bedroom and back.

Water the plant so that the soil remains moist in the pot—usually twice or thrice a week. This plant is not as hardy as the other two, and does require this little bit of care.

If you have followed all the tips in this book, and even after 8 hours of sleep, wake up tired and irritable, having these plants in your bedroom may do the trick for you. The tiredness could well be because of carbon dioxide build up through the night. Get these plants in your bedroom and all night long they will work hard, replenishing the oxygen in your space as you sleep. You will thank them each morning, when you wake up bright-eyed and smiling instead of feeling prickly and worn out.

Ideally, you should have a total of seven of these plants (in any combination you like) per person sleeping in your bedroom. Each of the plants should be at least a foot high or more to be able to create the oxygen that is required in the bedroom at night.

In my experience, though, even having three or four of them in the room is great. Better than having none at all. When you are planning a bedroom makeover, plan to have as many of these lovely plants in your room as possible.

A Shopping Guide

When we gave our book out for initial reviews, one of the most requested chapters to put in was a shopping list. People repeatedly told us, 'You have done so much research and spent so much money. Save your readers from wasting their time, effort and money and tell them what you found worked best for your bedroom and created a better sleep experience.'

So, here is a shopping list of a few things that we feel would be great in any bedroom and would significantly improve sleep quality. Everything listed here will send all the right messages to your brain, enhancing your sleep quality, making you feel rested and rejuvenated when you awaken in the morning.

Note that when you shop using our code on some of the websites mentioned below, you will get a discount and we may get a small commission.

We keep an updated shopping guide on our website: www.booksbybnd.com/shopping.

Paint

Every few years, it's a great idea to get a fresh coat of paint in your bedroom. The only reason we didn't do this was that after the painting is done, you have to deal with that noxious paint smell for a few weeks. Most commercially available paints have a host of toxic chemicals in them, and breathing those fumes even for a few days can be quite detrimental to your health and well-being. After some online research, we stumbled upon an organic non-toxic paint company. We used paints from them and our bedroom looked great and smelt amazing.

In case you are thinking of getting your bedroom painted, then use an organic, non-toxic paint. These days the big players like Asian Paints (Nilaya Naturals), Berger Paints (Breathe Easy) and Kansai Nerolac offer an organic, non-toxic paint line. Smaller companies offer even more natural paints. Choose your colour theme from these and keep the colours elegant and muted—soft whites, beiges or delicate pastels are great for your sleep space.

I recently got my bedroom and hall repainted and it was a pleasure to work with **www.ashwinpatelstudios.com**. I highly recommend Ashwin for getting the interiors of your home redone. Check their website for their other services.

Lights

Lighting is important. Give top priority to dimmable soft yellow lighting to be installed in your bedroom. Don't stop there; have dimmable yellow lights installed in your bathroom and toilet as well.

A high-quality visual environment promotes feelings of well-being.

Proper lighting without glare or shadows can reduce eye fatigue and headaches.

A warm and pleasant ambience can improve mood.

Good lighting should be flexible enough to light a given area while other areas remain in relative darkness. The best play of light and shadows has more to do with the placement of fixtures than wattage or the number of bulbs.

Besides, as we saw in an earlier chapter, there should be minimal to no flicker.

IngeniaTech is a fantastic little company that looks at the smallest details, providing comfort and health through bespoke lighting design. Your bedroom will be transformed into a place of beauty, feeling cozier and more inviting than ever before. You can check out their work on this website: **www.ingeniatech.in**.

If you are a more DIY person, get advice from **www.ashwinpatelstudios.com/lights** to help you choose the best type of lighting for your home. Of course, they can create and implement the entire lighting solution for your living spaces.

Air Conditioning

Air conditioning is almost mandatory these days unless you live up in the Himalayas or some such exotic location. My personal preference for air conditioners is a toss-up between Mitsubushi and Daikin. Over the years we have been through many brands in different places, and somehow feel the room cools down most uniformly and quickly with either of these two.

Air

The most natural of all air purifiers, those three magical plants we talked about in the bedroom chapter, are a must in every bedroom that takes sleep seriously. The areca palm, the money plant and the snake plant are all quite easy to get from any good nursery in your city. Remember that you need seven fully grown plants per person in the room. Of course, if your bedroom is small and there is less space, then get in as many plants as possible. Even one is better than none. A simple Google search will allow you to even order them online.

In Bangalore, Make My Garden is my nursery of choice. If you live in the Garden City, then you can visit them at their nursery or simply order these plants online from their website: **www.makemygarden.com/bedroomplants**. On this website, you will get a discount if you enter 'greatsleep' when you checkout.

For Delhi and NCR, BreatheEasy Labs provides the most amazing plants—aesthetically pretty, fully grown and ready to infuse your bedroom with oxygen. You can order your plants from **www.breatheeasylabs.com/collections/indoor-plants** and enter the discount code 'greatsleep' when you check.

To take the air quality in your bedroom to another dimension, I would strongly suggest that you invest in a really good air purifier. I have personally spent tons of money on the cheaper ones and eventually junked them. I hit upon the holy grail of air purifiers—the IQAir Healthpro and Cleanroom lines.

These machines tick every single box that you can think of and are one of the best investments we have made for our bedroom. A room with an IQAir purifier in it feels as though you are somewhere up at a hill station, breathing wonderful, fresh air, utterly different from the stale city air most people are resigned to. IQAir is a Swiss–German appliance and you can buy it in India with warranty and guaranteed availability of replacement filters.

It is an expensive machine—costs between Rs 1.5–2.2 lakhs, depending on the model you choose—but don't let this price put you off. The tremendous improvement in air quality it brings to your sleeping space is well worth every penny you spend on it. Many friends who bought this on my recommendation reported less allergic reactions, dramatic reduction in breathing problems and, of course, much better sleep. You can get these amazing little monsters from **www.breatheeasylabs.com/collections/air-purifiers**—enter 'greatsleep' when you checkout, and you will get a discount on your purchase. I highly recommend BreatheEasy Labs machines. They have stellar after-sales service, are quick, efficient and courteous and a pleasure to do business with.

Speakers

I am quite an audiophile and love to have a good speaker setup in my bedroom to listen to soft soothing music or some chanting at night. My personal favourite speaker is the Triangle AIO. It costs a pretty penny, but the sound quality at that price range is phenomenal. You can buy it from **www.yoursmusically.com/wirelessspeakers** and entering the code 'greatsleep' will get you a discount when you order from this website.

Curtains

If you live in an apartment or a house in a city, then blackout curtains to create that beautiful velvety darkness in your bedroom need to be on the top of your shopping list. There will always be a pesky street light, or a neighbour's light that will want to shine through your window and mess up your sleep. You will need to get your blackout curtains made to order from a specialty curtain shop. Ashwin's website has a whole gamut of options for creating your blackout curtains. Check **www.ashwinpatelstudios.com/curtains** for details. Use the code 'greatsleep' when you checkout for a discount on your purchase. They ship all over India.

Bed Clothes

My favourite bedtime clothes are from the BYogi Vishraam line. Luxurious, pure, soft cotton clothes in white and a few beautiful pastel shades, make these garments just perfect for sleep. They are comfortably chic and can even double up as loungewear, though they do crumple a bit. The clothes are light and the fabric lets you breathe. These are easy to wear, hassle-free garments. You can get them on this website: **www.byogi.store/vishraam.**

For the readers of this book, they have a special deal on their entire Vishraam range. Enter 'greatsleep' on checkout to get a discount on whatever you have shopped for from their website.

The Mattress, Pillows and Bed Linen

Your mattress itself is of paramount importance and it's best to have something that you truly enjoy sleeping on. Mattresses can be extremely expensive and it would be a great idea to buy them from a shop that allows you to sleep on their mattress for a few days to test them out.

I whole heartedly recommend the mattresses from PEPS India. These mattresses check all the boxes about what truly great mattresses should be like—firm, yet comfortable and made are from the best quality material possible. There are absolutely no corners cut in their manufacture. My favourites from the PEPS India range are SpineGuard, Organica and Restonic. They make nice pillows as well—my favourite is the Neck Guard Memory Moulded Pillow—Contour. You can buy the mattresses and pillows along with other bed friendly products from their website **www.pepsindia.com**—use the discount code 'greatsleep' on checkout. They deliver across India.

As a cheaper alternative, the local gadda-walas make pretty good mattresses and pillows—tell them to use the best quality cotton that they can source for the stuffing.

Bed linen is a personal preference. Sleep research says that white sheets are the best for great sleep. I find white too plain and prefer simple and elegant floral or paisley patterns on my bedsheets. You see what feels best for you and get that. Ensure the bed sheets are made of the best quality cotton and have a high thread count. Avoid synthetic stuff like polyester—even though you may get much better durability if it's mixed in. Good bedsheets can make you feel like you are sleeping on a cloud.

Skin Care

After your hot shower and before you are ready to hit the bed, some skin pampering feels just wonderful. One of my very favourite brands is Shankara.

Shankara has been creating all-natural beauty and wellness products, handcrafted to the highest standards. Their offerings nourish the body, mind and spirit. They blend ancient super herbs with modern actives to sustainably create 100% natural and result-oriented skincare products.

A night skin care routine helps you let go of the stress of the day and recharge so you can look your best for tomorrow.

My three-step night routine by Shankara:

Step 1
Hydrating cleanser: This is an ultra-soothing and gentle cleanser that leaves the skin feeling soft and supple with the combination of chamomile, lavender, neem and calendula.

Step 2
Brightening serum: This helps counter the effects of pollution with just a few drops of usage. Reduce ruddiness

and discolouration, even and lighten skin tone, and uncover a more radiant you.
Or
Rose water: A few spritzes of high quality rose water works wonders on your skin. Remember to let it dry out naturally before moving to Step 3.

Step 3
Kumkumadi oil: This is a miracle skin tonic that is light, absorbs easily and will nourish, rejuvenate and firm the skin while reducing discoloration and blemishes.

Go through this fantastic little ritual and let all those lovely herbs work all night through on your face. When you wake up in the morning, your face will be aglow. You can buy some of India's finest natural beauty products from **www.shankara.in**. For your night ritual kit, beautifully packed in a specially designed pouch, go directly to **www.shankara.in/nightglow**. Enter 'greatsleep' when you checkout for a great discount on anything you buy from the Shankara website.

Vacuum Cleaner

A good powerful vacuum cleaner is another fabulous addition to your enhanced sleep arsenal. Vacuuming your bed linen and the mattress at least once or twice a week will get rid of pesky dust mites. Vacuuming down your curtains regularly helps reduce the allergens in your room as well. This will help you sleep better as your immune system doesn't have to deal with microscopic allergens while you slumber. My favourite brand? Dyson.

Candles

One set of little accessories I love to have in my bedroom are candles. Make sure you get the unscented ones, or if you like fragrances, something with a subtle fragrance like rose or jasmine. Small tea lights to designer candles all look really pretty in the night and bring a beautiful warm glow to your bedroom.

Amber Glasses

We have talked at length about the effects of exposure to white and blue light after sunset on sleep quality. There are times when you simply cannot avoid these lights. The easiest solution is to get blue light blocking glasses—they are typically amber or rose tinted, and do a fabulous job of almost eliminating blue and white light from hitting your eyes. As a bonus, they turned out to be great conversation starters as well.

Visit your local optician and ask them to make these specifically for you.

Grounding Mats

I cannot overemphasise the benefits of earthing or grounding—we talked about this in the chapter on the art of waking up. The benefits of being barefoot on the earth are almost magical, yet most people end up not finding the time to do it. They then have to deal with inflammation and all its associated aches, pains and woes.

I was delighted to find a small startup company right here in India that makes grounding mats. These are simple yet effective solutions to get more than 90% of the benefit of being barefoot on the earth, right from your desk in the office to your home. I have been personally using grounding mats for over a year now and can vouch for the tremendous health benefits they have given me.

Grounding bedsheets allow you to stay grounded for the entire 8 hours that you sleep through the night, compounding the awesome effects of being grounded. These products could perhaps be the simplest, fastest way to better health and are totally worth investing in.

Get these grounding products from **www.groundingindia.com** and you can get a discount when you order by entering the code 'greatsleep'.

As mentioned earlier, we keep an updated shopping list on our website: **www.booksbybnd.com/sys/media.**

Sri Sri Ravi Shankar

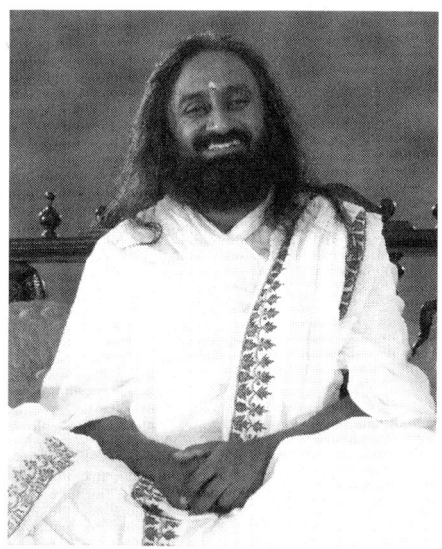

Gurudev Sri Sri Ravi Shankar is a universally revered spiritual and humanitarian leader. His vision of a violence-and stress-free society through the reawakening of human values has inspired millions to broaden their spheres of responsibility and work towards the betterment of the world.

He is a multifaceted social visionary whose initiatives include conflict resolution, disaster and trauma relief, poverty alleviation, women empowerment, prisoner rehabilitation, education for all and campaigns against female foeticide and child labour. He is engaged in peace negotiations and counselling in conflict zones around the world.

In 1981, he established The Art of Living Foundation, an educational and humanitarian non-governmental organisation. In 1997, Gurudev founded the International Association for Human Values (IAHV) to lead sustainable development projects. He is also a co-founder of India Against Corruption (IAC).

He has reached out to many millions of people worldwide through personal interactions, public events, teachings, Art of Living workshops and humanitarian initiatives. He has brought to the masses ancient practices that were traditionally kept exclusive, and has designed many self-development techniques that can be easily integrated into daily life to calm the mind and instill confidence and enthusiasm in people. One of Gurudev's most unique offerings to the world is the Sudarshan Kriya, a powerful breathing technique that facilitates physical, mental, emotional and social well-being.

Gurudev has received numerous accolades, including the highest civilian awards of Colombia, Mongolia and Paraguay. In 2016, he was conferred the Padma Vibhushan, one of the highest civilian awards of India. He has addressed several international forums, including TED 2010 at Monterey, the United Nations Millennium World Peace Summit (2000), the World Economic Forum (2001, 2003) and several parliaments across the globe.

Gurudev travels to nearly 40 countries every year, exemplifying his call to globalise wisdom.

His universal and simple message is that love and wisdom can prevail over hatred and distress.

Read more about Gurudev, find out about His tour schedule as well as His latest spiritual knowledge and meditation discourses from **www.srisriravishankar.org**.

The Art of Living Foundation Courses

It's a well-established scientific fact that happy people are more productive, creative, efficient and effective. Who wouldn't want all this and more in their lives? Gift yourself this happiness advantage by engaging with Art of Living's various programmes for individuals and communities.

And if you are thinking, *But I am already happy,* ... surely you are not allergic to more happiness, right?

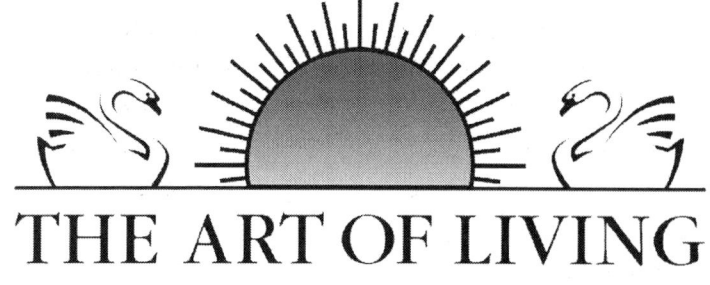

The Meditation and Breath Workshop

Weight gain (or loss) without a diet change, hair fall, stomachache and stomach disorders, forgetfulness, sleep disorders, headaches, frequent colds, high or low blood pressure and infections are only a few symptoms of stress.

Most people just accept stress and tension as an inevitable part of their lives. They feel that they simply have to 'cope' with the problems associated with stress and get on with life.

The Art of Living Meditation and Breath Workshop includes techniques that allow you to de-stress and live your life without all the associated distress.

Positive psychology is a powerful new branch of mental health founded on the belief that people want to lead meaningful and fulfilling lives to cultivate what is best within themselves and to enhance their experiences of love, work and play. The Art of Living courses feature yoga, meditation and other interactive processes that allow you to do exactly that.

The profound and powerful Sudarshan Kriya that is taught in the Meditation and Breath Workshop enables you to effortlessly let go of your stresses and tensions and introduces within you a tranquillity you never knew existed.

You can be what you have always wanted to be: healthy, poised, calm, relaxed and confident.

For courses taught by Khurshed, Dinesh and their team, go to www.inergyworld.com and click on the Schedules tab.

The Sleep and Anxiety Relief Workshop

During the unprecedented troubled times of the Covid-19 pandemic, millions of people all over the world developed all sorts of phobias and fears. Among all the other things that went awry, this compounded the problem of compromised sleep and a lot of lives spiralled downwards.

The Sleep and Anxiety Relief workshop has specific protocols to deal with anxiety and panic. Powerful yoga sequences, delicate pranayamas and specialised mudras are taught and perfected during the workshop, bringing tremendous relief to the participants.

The profound and potent Sudarshan Kriya forms a core part of this workshop. Practising it brings about a sense of deep relaxation and calm within oneself. People feel ready once more to face the challenges that life throws at them, and slowly gain confidence as they begin to piece their life back together. Hope is kindled as people learn to smile from the heart once again.

You will find schedules of courses taught by Khurshed, Dinesh and their team, and more details about this programme on **www.inergyworld.com**.

The YES!+ Programme

Anyone who is twelve or thirteen can't wait to be eighteen. A thirty-five or forty-year-old yearns for his youth. Everyone wants to be eighteen, except for the ones who *are* eighteen!

The age group eighteen to thirty is a wonderful time in life. You feel you can do absolutely anything—that you can conquer the world! Your body and mind are at their peak. Unfortunately, so is the confusion. There are too many options and challenges. To top it off, you have raging hormones. Things you do or don't in this period can profoundly affect the rest of your life.

You desperately need a calm, poised mind to be able to take sensible decisions. The YES!+ course was created by me and Dinesh under the guidance of Gurudev Sri Sri Ravi Shankar to address all these issues and more.

The course sparkles with dialogue, is peppered with fun and humour and liberally sprinkled with insightful interactive processes. This allows our participants to explore a dimension of the mind most people don't even know exist. This course is a delectable treat for a young person who is going places.

The Sudarshan Kriya is taught during this course, along with a few other techniques, to enhance focus and concentration levels.

You will have the tools and the ability to be able to live the life you *want* to live instead of the life you *have* to live.

Sahaj Samadhi Meditation

Everyone has experienced a meditative state in moments of deep joy, or when completely engrossed in an activity—the mind becomes still, light and is at ease for just a few moments. Almost all of us have sporadically experienced such moments of utter calm and peace, but we are unable to repeat them at will.

The Sahaj Samadhi Meditation programme teaches you how. This technique almost instantly alleviates the practitioner from stress-related problems, deeply relaxes the mind and rejuvenates the system.

'Sahaj' is a Sanskrit word that means natural or effortless. 'Samadhi' is a deep, blissful, meditative state. 'Sahaj Samadhi Meditation', hence, is a natural, effortless system of meditation.

Regular practice of the technique can transform the quality of one's life by culturing the system to maintain the peace, energy and expanded awareness throughout the day.

Khurshed and Dinesh teach this sublime course once every month or two. Enrol for their next Sahaj Samadhi Meditation course through **www.inergyworld.com**.

The Advanced Meditation Course (AMC)

The AMC is a four to ten day residential silence programme. It begins early in the morning with yoga and Sudarshan Kriya, has guided meditation sessions through the day and ends with blissful chanting and knowledge sessions by Gurudev in the evening. Tasty, healthy food is served to all course participants at meal times.

The course helps you recharge and rejuvenate yourself so that you are better equipped to respond with equanimity and poise to the stresses and challenges that contemporary life throws at you. It is an intensive work over for the mind and body. People who have undergone this course report feeling refreshed, their faces aglow and their hearts at peace.

After almost three decades of practising meditation, Dinesh and I still attend one AMC every year, and we recommend that you do too. Take a few days off, unplug yourself from the world and totally relax.

Though AMCs are now conducted in cities and towns all over the world, we feel the best way to get the most out of them is to go do them at one of Art of Living's many ashrams.

Our favourite places to do an AMC? The Art of Living ashrams in Bangalore, Rishikesh, Gujarat, Germany, the US and Canada.

Khurshed and Dinesh facilitate this amazing course five or six times each year, usually in Rishikesh, in an ashram located on the banks of the magical Ganga. Most times, weather permitting, the entire course goes white water rafting on the Ganga. Join them in Rishikesh for an adventure on the inside as well the outside. Find details about the courses they teach on **www.inergyworld.com**.

Yogic Fitness

An Introduction to Holistic Health and Fitness

Congratulations! You have a body. Not just *any* body—a human body. It can be very easy to take this for granted.

It has taken many millennia for our bodies to evolve into the astounding pieces of super complex organic technology that they are. We experience life through them. For an optimal experience of our time on the planet, we need to ensure that our bodies stay fit and healthy. Disease happens when we forget this.

Time, money and effort invested in building robust good health will not then be wasted being ill, staring at ceilings and feeling miserable.

Yogic Fitness (YF) is a unique programme that starts you off on that most precious journey: great health!

In three sessions of three to four hours each, you will be introduced to the art and science of health, strength and fitness.

YF brings together three elements required for vibrant good health: exercise, diet and rest.

You will be taught foundation exercises that will get your body moving the way it has been designed to.

Diet can be a game changer when it comes to fitness. Knowledge of what to eat, what not to eat and why to eat or not eat something is paramount for success. You will learn the basics, enough to whet your appetite. Besides, you will be served a fantastic meal in class each day.

The critical importance of rest will be explained—the why and how of sleep, along with an introduction to meditation. Each session will end with deeply relaxing stillness.

Continue your journey online. All exercises taught and full-body workouts based on the exercises you have learned will be available for you to view online, so you can refresh and fine-tune what you learned in class.

Enrol in the Yogic Fitness course to experience the magic of great health for yourself. You will find more details on **www.inergyworld.com**.

The Divya Samaj ka Nirman (DSN) Course

There are rivers to cross and mountains to climb ... but the biggest mountains are mostly the mountains in our own minds.

The DSN is an evening and three full action-packed days of learning about our self-imposed limitations and breaking them. It is an emotional, physical and spiritual roller-coaster ride, an exciting challenge for the courageous and an inspiration for the ones who want to be inspired.

All of us have good intentions and fantastic ideas for ourselves, our families and friends, and for society. Regrettably, these good intentions hardly ever translate into action. These wonderful ideas remain as ideas and frequently we are forced to compromise on our dreams and ambitions.

The mind stuff disempowers us and doesn't allow us to lead the life we are born to live. It buries us in the humdrum and the mundane and keeps us from reaching for the stars. It is quite a journey to get rid of these limitations, and the DSN programme provides a fantastic start.

The DSN overflows with knowledge sessions, group discussions, games, advanced yoga techniques such as Padmasadhana and many chances to go out into the world and make a difference during the course itself. The DSN experience will leave you enriched and empowered.

Discover your inner superhero and start to live the life you have always dreamt about.

There are many other courses that Art of Living offers, from learning yoga to vegetarian cooking and almost everything in between.

The teachers and volunteers of the Art of Living Foundation strive to create a better world for themselves and their communities through various services like planting trees, rejuvenating rivers, running free schools in villages and slums, empowering women, providing vocational training for village youth, helping disaster victims, and more. You can find descriptions and details of all this and more on **www.artofliving.org**.

Art of Living Workshops Online

The Meditation and Breath Workshop, The Sleep and Anxiety Relief Workshop, Sahaj Samadhi Meditation Course and the Advanced Meditation Programme are all offered as online courses as well. Course schedules, more details about these course and other Art of Living courses that are taught by Khurshed (Bawa), Dinesh and their team are on **www.inergyworld.com**.

Integrated Craniosacral Therapy

Craniosacral Therapy (CST) is a profound, non-invasive, healing process that works through gentle touch to release stress, disturbance, injury and deep-seated trauma. It is known to benefit an entire range of problems, from minor aches and pains to severe chronic conditions.

It restores balance across the various systems of the body–mind system, transforming it back to a state of vibrant health. And for those who are healthy, it boosts all the systems of the body, bringing another level of well-being within them.

Many times we abuse our body by disrupting its natural rhythms (not sleeping or eating on time), overindulging (eating wrong types of food, working too hard, not sleeping enough, etc.) and consuming obvious poisons like alcohol, tobacco or recreational drugs, causing it terrible stress. Accidents, bugs, illnesses and other mishaps also contribute to the assault on it.

The body is a brilliant piece of engineering and most times manages to bounce back to health, albeit, with a little bit of leftover distress. These distresses pile up over time, causing our immune systems to break down, and this creates disease.

However, there is a vast intelligence in the body and almost infinite resources available, if only you could tap into them. Craniosacral Therapy acts as a catalyst for you to tap into your own system, use resources available to you and create great health. Of course, lifestyle changes would need to happen alongside CST for it to have a more dramatic, permanent effect.

Through touch, a skilled therapist can figure out what's wrong in it and bring about balance and harmony in the body by supplementing its own drive towards great health.

Khurshed (Bawa), Dinesh and Dr Ankita Dhelia have created a flagship in-depth training of eight seminars of five to seven days, spread over approximately twenty months, for Sri Sri Tattva Centre of Healing Arts. The great news is that you don't need any medical background to undergo this training. Almost anyone without serious health conditions can do it. Our youngest student is just eighteen years of age and oldest so far is seventy-six!

Our entire series of seminars is designed to nurture and enable you to become a confident, competent, compassionate and effective integrated craniosacral therapist. CST is more than a century old and has a rich legacy of techniques and literature. You will be exposed to key concepts and the correct protocols of this technique which will lay a strong foundation for you to grow in this exciting field.

We believe that CST is a unique combination of technical knowledge of the human body and spiritual practices in action. To succeed as a therapist, you will need knowledge of human anatomy, cultivate body awareness and develop the ability to meditate. All these aspects form a core part of our training.

Our training is mainly based on the classical texts of Osteopathy and Craniosacral Therapy written by Dr Andrew

Taylor Still, Dr William Sutherland, Dr Harold Magoun, Dr T.M. Littlejohn and Dr Rollin Becker. We have referred to texts by Michael Kern, Franklyn Sills, Cherionna Menzan-Sills, Roger Gilchrist, Hugh Milne and Thomas Atlee as well.

This knowledge is expertly woven in with the philosophy and techniques of Indian spirituality, inspired by Gurudev Sri Sri Ravi Shankar, to create a one-of-a-kind learning experience for our students. We are the only school in the world offering a programme like this.

We extend a warm welcome to you to undergo this training and create vibrant health for yourself and others. Many people opt to become CST practitioners to supplement their income. Quite a few of our students have made it their full-time career.

And just in case you are wondering if CST can help heal fractured sleep ... the answer is a resounding yes! We have helped scores of people sleep better through CST treatments.

We start a few new batches every year. To know more about Craniosacral Therapy and our training schedules, please check out **www.sstcha.com/**.

To apply for this training, please visit **www.sstcha.com/**.

Dinesh and I give private CST sessions as well—please write to **khurshedcst@gmail.com** to book an appointment.

Workshops with Khurshed and Dinesh

Bach Flower Remedies

Almost a century ago, Dr Edward Bach discovered that certain flowers in nature have the ability to affect our emotions positively. His original Bach Flower system of 38 remedies and their combinations are easy for anyone to understand and use. Using the 38 remedies in their permutations and combinations, you would be able to handle over two million states of mind.

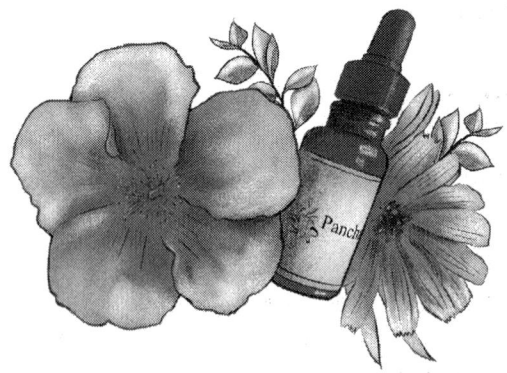

The Bach Flower Remedies can work in conjunction with herbs, Homeopathy and any other medication. They are safe for everyone, including children, pregnant women, the elderly, pets and even plants.

I have had almost a decade of experience in using them. The refrain I hear most often from my clients is: 'I feel I am myself again.'

Of course, sleep becomes deeper and more restful when we can figure out a relevant personal mix and you regularly partake of it. And as we have seen throughout this book, when sleep is fixed, a lot of other things get fixed as well.

Over and over again, I have seen that the mind can be the biggest obstacle to your success. When the storms of emotions subside, you get the ability to think clearly and act rationally. Success comes faster and easier. The Bach Flower Remedies complement everything we have talked about in this book extremely well.

You can book a private consultation with me through my website, **www.bachflowers.in**.

If you wish, you can learn about these amazing remedies through a series of trainings certified by the Bach Centre UK. I am a registered Bach Flower practitioner and a certified Level 1 and 2 trainer with the Bach Centre, UK.

Bach Flower Remedies Training Programmes

The Bach Flower remedies are loosely based on homeopathic principles and the remedies are simple, though not simplistic. Anyone, anywhere can learn about them and benefit from their gentle healing properties. The Bach Centre UK has created three levels to learn about the remedies.

Here is a snapshot of the topics covered in the first two levels that I am certified to teach:

- Overview of the 38 remedies
- Subtle differences between similar remedies
- Remedy making and dosage
- Mood and type remedies
- Essence and relevance of Dr Bach's philosophy
- Gain confidence to create personal mixes of the remedies for yourself, friends and family

- Fun and interactive group activities
- Stories and personal anecdotes
- Detailed class notes for self-paced studying
- Certification from the Bach Centre UK

I am glad to extend a personal invitation to you to enrol in these programmes and learn about the Bach Flower System with me.

There is a lot to cover in the Level 1 programme and it is jam-packed with interesting material. I integrate Adult Learning Theory and principles of NLP into my training so that the vast subject matter becomes easily accessible to all my students—and they can effortlessly remember nuances and details.

The Level 2 programme is an introspective and leisurely journey. You will have plenty of time to think about which remedy mix could be the most relevant for you and your friends and families. You will gain confidence in the system as you understand how to differentiate between remedies that may sound similar in their application.

A typical class can have lectures, question-and-answer sessions, group interactive processes, fun challenges and more. Detailed class notes are given for each session, so you can refer to them at a later date and even continue to learn at your own pace. You will have crystal-clear instructions about how to integrate this almost magical system into your life by the end of the two programmes.

I offer both online as well as live classes for the Level 1 and 2 programmes.

The online and live version of the Level 1 programme is conducted over 4 sessions of about three hours each.

The live version of the Level 2 programme consists of 4-5 sessions of 3-4 hours each. The online version is 6 sessions of

3 hours each, typically spread over 6-7 weeks. For the online version, you will need to complete and submit a dossier that you will get access to from the Bach Centre website.

You can find more details about the remedies, these workshops and their schedules on my website, **www.bachflowers.in**.

The third and last level certifies you as a practitioner—the Bach Centre offers online as well as offline courses for Level 3. You can find more details on **www.bachcentre.com**.

I hope to be a Level 3 teacher by the end of 2022.

THE POWER OF SLEEP

The Power of Sleep Workshop is designed to be a systematic way to engineer better sleep. We have methodically drawn on all the knowledge we have about sleep, then added in our own personal experience to create a unique way to sleep better. You can learn an almost foolproof go-to-sleep and wake-up ritual step-by-baby-step during the course of this workshop. Following the protocols you will learn will ensure you feel deeply rested and rejuvenated. You will have learned to harness the power of sleep to help you achieve your dreams.

You will have access to a set of pre-recorded online videos which will let you learn and implement the best practices about sleep at your own pace. Periodically, all our students will be invited to a live online question-and-answer session with Dinesh and me—so if you have any doubts or questions around the subject of sleep, we can answer them.

This workshop supplements all you have read about sleep in this book and builds on it to allow you to sleep the way nature intended. We will be constantly adding more content to the workshop as we learn more and more about sleep. You will have access to all the question-and-answer sessions on sleep that have been recorded as well.*

Within a few weeks, you will be able to reap all the glorious benefits of great sleep—and we truly hope you will be able to *Sleep Your Way to Success*.

Please visit **www.booksbybnd.com/workshops/powerofsleep** for more details.

---

*This workshop is not for people suffering from any clinical sleep-related problems like sleep apnea. They may derive some sort of benefit, but may continue to require medical intervention. This workshop is for normal people who wished they slept better.

Study Sutras

*'Everyone used to tell me to use my brain.
No one told me exactly how to do it.'*

You could be a student working your way through university, a professional struggling with new concepts you have to study or someone who is simply curious and wants to know more.

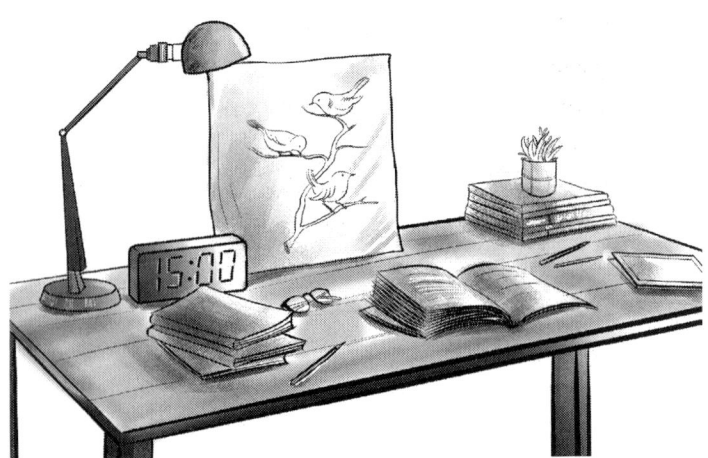

Our brain is a super advanced piece of organic technology. Unfortunately, we inherited it without a user manual. Study Sutras is a three-hour, fast-paced workshop delving into the intricacies of how to make the brain work with dazzling efficiency.

This workshop, which is based on a few chapters from the book, *Ready, Study, Go!: Smart Ways to Learn*, will create a paradigm shift in the way you learn. It will make the process of studying efficient, enjoyable and more meaningful. It will transform the way you think and possibly even the way you live.

Facts about the brain, study tips, brain hacks and, if time permits, a guided meditation await you in this workshop designed by Dinesh and me.

Do read our book. It is available online and offline, at bookstores around the world. With tips and techniques to make studying an intriguing activity, it has sold more than 50,000 copies.

For more about the book, visit **www.bawandinesh.in/ready-study-go/**.

To buy it from amazon.in, follow this link: **bit.ly/readystudygo**.

To get it from amazon.com, go here: **bit.ly/readystudygointl**.

Note: In some countries, our workshop, Study Sutras, is called Study Smart.

We will be offering an online version of this workshop soon. Visit **www.booksbybnd.com/workshops/studysutras** for more information.

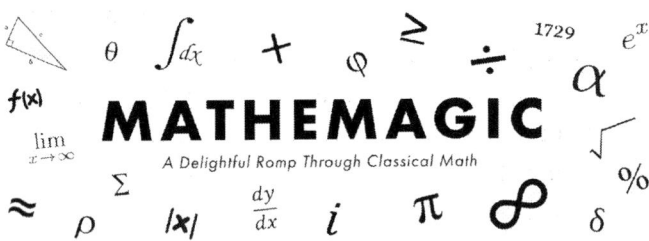

MATHEMAGIC
A Delightful Romp Through Classical Math

'I hate math' is a familiar refrain. Studying math, for most people, is usually an exercise in frustration; for some, even terror. This is largely because of a lack of interest in the subject, which is compounded by uninspiring teachers and insipid prescribed textbooks that utterly malign the subject.

There is hardly any life without math. Math pervades all we do, yet most people are repelled by it. This is sad, because Mathematics is a subject of magic and exquisite beauty. We had had enough of people berating this lovely subject and decided to do something about it.

We put together a workshop that would primarily eliminate the almost irrational fear that many people have of the subject, as well as effortlessly reveal its intrinsic beauty.

Starting with some frivolous playing around with numbers and multiplication, the workshop quickly moves on to cover some of the basics of real analysis, calculus, number theory and finite mathematics. We focus on fundamental concepts and reveal the elegant logic that hides behind rigorous mathematical proofs. A few fascinating stories from the history of math and mathematicians are woven into the material.

The entire workshop is peppered with healthy doses of humour as well as a few interactive exercises for the participants, so that they can discover the joy of applying logic to solve problems for themselves.

Initially Dinesh and I taught the workshop ourselves, but owing to increased demand, we now have a number of trained and talented teachers besides us. Through this workshop, you too will feel the passion and love that we have for math.

Mathemagic has been designed to be a thoroughly entertaining two-hour learning experience, a delightful foray into the basics of some fairly advanced math.

We will soon be offering Mathemagic as an online workshop. Visit **www.booksbybnd.com/workshops/mathemagic** for more information.

Bibliography

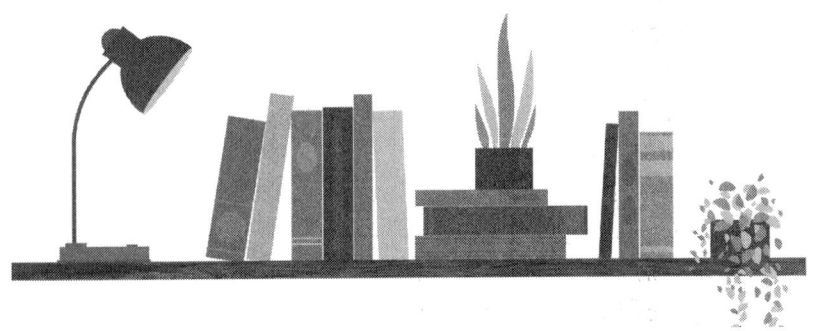

Sleep

There are many books on sleep out there. I found these to be the best reads. Mathew Walker is highly recommended, for even more in-depth science about sleep and dreaming.
1. *Why We Sleep* – Mathew Walker
2. *The Sleep Revolution* – Arianna Huffington
3. *The Sleep Solution: Why Your Sleep Is Broken and How to Fix It* – W. Chris Winter
4. *Say Goodnight to Insomnia* – Gregg D. Jacobs

In addition to these, I am also intrigued by the work of Dr Sasha Gominak. She believes that any sort of sleep disorder can be sorted out by taking the right types of vitamin supplements. I have not had the opportunity to experience or evaluate any of it, but if you are curious, head over to **www.drgominak.com/** to check out what she talks about.

Success

There are many, many great books on success. I list here some of my personal favourites—ones that have influenced my thinking and my life. You might find shades of all these books reflected in what I write when I talk about success.

In *Atomic Habits,* James Clear talks about how small actions, done over time, can generate big results. A book on how to develop and sustain great habits and kick bad habits. It's a great read.

Through captivating little anecdotes, Morgan Housel talks about how doing well with money is not so much about what you know about finances, but more about how you behave. What could be the relationship between an ice age and becoming as rich as Warren Buffet? Or how did a janitor in a small town in the US have $8 million? Read *The Psychology of Money* and find out.

If you have ever wondered about what is Neuro-linguistic programming (NLP), then *Introducing NLP* by Joseph O'Connor and John Seymour is the book for you. Be warned, though, unless you have done a seminar or two on NLP, this book will be a difficult read.

About 77% of leaders think they do a good job of engaging their people, yet 88% of employees say their leaders don't engage enough. There is also a high level of suffering in the workplace: 35% of employees would forgo a pay raise to see their boss fired. How leaders think—and how they should think and what would happen if they did—all of it is in this brilliant book, *The Mind of a Leader* by Rasmus Hougaard and Jacqueline Carter.

Creating great conversations is an art and a science and this is explored in Judith Glaser's book, *Conversational Intelligence.*

Rich Dad Poor Dad by Robert Kiyosaki is about handling money and your relationship with money. It is the story of growing up with two dads—his real father and the father of his best friend, his rich dad—and the ways in which both men shaped his thoughts about money and investing. The book explodes the myth that you need to earn a high income to be rich and explains the difference between working for money and having your money work for you. If you do pick up this book, don't bother reading any of Kiyosaki's other books. They all say the exact same thing in many different ways.

Superbetter is one of my favourite books. Jane McGonigal, the writer, is a gamer. The book is all about how she gamified her life to come out of a serious concussion which left her wanting to die. The system she created for herself called 'superbetter', has helped thousands around the world.

1. *Atomic Habits* – James Clear
2. *The Psychology of Money* – Morgan Housel
3. *Introducing NLP* – Joseph O'Connor and John Seymour
4. *The Mind of a Leader* – Rasmus Hougaard and Jacqueline Carter
5. *Conversational Intelligence* – Judith E. Glaser
6. *Rich Dad, Poor Dad* – Robert Kiyosaki
7. *Superbetter* – Jane McGonigal

Happiness

Our book, *Ready Study Go!*, is about learning how to learn—but it doesn't end there. This warm, funny book explores the many obstacles that you might face when you sit down to learn something—from empty wallets to broken hearts, and a lot of stuff in between. It will show you how learning new things can be fun—and can make you happy!

Happiness Express is all about living better. We explore the various aspects of life that make happiness an even more integral part of your life than ever before.

Shawn Achor's and Emma Seppala's books talk about the science of happiness and positive psychology and list the steps to achieve it.

1. *Ready Study Go!* – Khurshed Batliwala and Dinesh Ghodke
2. *Happiness Express* – Khurshed Batliwala and Dinesh Ghodke
3. *The Happiness Advantage* – Shawn Achor
4. *The Happiness Track* – Emma Seppala

Meditation

Everyone should read all these books again and again throughout their lives. They will enrich you beyond measure.

1. *An Intimate Note to the Sincere Seeker* – Sri Sri Ravi Shankar
2. *Commentary on the Yoga Sutras of Patanjali* – Sri Sri Ravi Shankar
3. *Gurudev: On the Plateau of the Peak* – Bhanumati Narasimhan
4. *Yoga Vasishtha* – Swami Venkateshanada
5. *Srimad Bhagavad Gita* – Gita Press

Food

The first two books listed below are enjoyable reads about why you should eat vegetarian food and what happens to food once you put it in your mouth.

The other books are my favourite recipe books. Some have non-vegetarian recipes in them, but with a bit of jugglery these recipes can be made vegetarian. Vidhu

Mittal's book is outstanding for Indian food and Niloufer's passion for food and cooking, especially Parsi recipes, is evident on every page.

I own quite a few of Jamie Oliver's books. I enjoy his style and his recipes. His book of Italian recipes is my most favourite.

The Moosewood Cookbook has many interesting recipes to experiment with. *Oh She Glows* is an exclusively vegan cookbook, one of the finest I have for vegan recipes.

1. *Food Revolution* – John Robbins
2. *Gut: The Inside Story Of Our Body's Most Underrated Organ* – Guila Enders
3. *Pure and Simple* – Vidhu Mittal
4. *My Bombay Kitchen* – Niloufer Ichaporia King
5. *Jamie's Italy* – Jamie Oliver
6. *The New Moosewood Cookbook* – Mollie Katzen
7. *The Oh She Glows Cookbook* – Angela Liddon

Exercise

These books are for reference only. Please don't try to learn exercises from a book. Get a good personal trainer. You run the risk of seriously injuring yourself if you exercise without a trainer at least to begin with.

1. *Men's Health Big Book of Exercises* – Adam Campbell
2. *Women's Health Big Book of Exercises* – Adam Campbell
3. *Starting Strength*, (third edition) – Mark Rippetoe

Bach Flower Remedies

Dr Edward Bach's book, *The 12 Healers*, is available as a free download from the Bach Center website— **www.bachcentre.com** and is a superb introduction to his system. The Bach Centre website and my own

www.bachflowers.in have many additional resources for learning about the remedies as well as details about courses that can certify you to be a Bach practitioner.

Over the years, various practitioners have found Dr Bach's original book to be quite terse, and have written books of their own to augment his work. My favourite three among the scores of books I have read on the subject are listed below:
1. *Emotional Wisdom with the Bach Flower Remedies* – Lynn Macwhinnie
2. *Bach Flower Therapy: Theory and Practice* – Mechthild Scheffer
3. *The Healing Herbs of Edward Bach* – Julian and Martine Barnard

Other Related Interesting Reads

We touched briefly upon the subject of earthing in the 'Waking Up' chapter. Clinton Ober, the guy who 'discovered' earthing, talks about his subject with passion and simplicity. He will have you walking barefoot in the grass before you are even halfway through the book.

As you are reading this sentence, you are breathing. And there is nothing truly more important than the act of breathing. Breath is life itself. James Nestor, in his book *Breath: The New Science of a Lost Art,* talks about how we humans as a species are breathing wrong, twenty-five thousand times a day, and the grave consequences of it. He suggests various breathing techniques through this fantastically researched book that could help correct our breathing and hence our health and well-being.

Emotional Freedom Technique (EFT) works really well for people with sleep problems among many other health conditions. It's all about tapping gently on various points of power on the body to bring it back towards health. Nick has written a great book (*The Tapping Solution*) on the topic and you will not need to read any other on the subject of EFT.

The Circadian Code starts really well, but then drags on and on ... However, it has a lot of information about the 'when'—from exercise to sleeping and everything in between.

Douglas Adams' book (*Last Chance to See*) on the dangerous threats that our environment is facing is alarming and funny at the same time. It's a must-read.

Mitch Albom writes exquisitely and this is a magical chronicle of the time he spends with his mentor from twenty years ago, through which he shares Morrie's lasting gift with the world (*Tuesdays with Morrie*).

On a Wing and a Prayer: Spirituality for the Reluctant, the Curious and the Seeker by Kushal Choksi is a riveting read. He was in the twin towers on 9/11. He survived. Everything he had done till then as a Wall Street trader with Goldman Sachs felt meaningless. He felt a void within him that nothing could fill. Then, reluctantly, he decided to spend an afternoon with a spiritual master in New York City. This is a warm, funny, hopeful and charming read. You will love it!

No reading list by me would be complete without a few books from my all-time favourite author, P.G. Wodehouse. His hilarious stories from Blandings Caste, involving the ninth Earl of Emsworth, his sister Connie and his beloved pig, the Empress of Blandings, will leave you rolling on the floor laughing. There are always impostors who need to be exposed and broken hearts that need repairing at Blandings ...

Bibliography

1. *Earthing* – Clinton Ober, Stephen Sinatra, Martin Zucker
2. *Breath: The New Science of a Lost Art* – James Nestor
3. *Ayurveda Simplified* – Dr Nisha Manikandan
4. *Ayurveda and Panchakarma: The Science of Healing and Rejuvenation* – Sunil V. Joshi
5. *Ayurveda: The Science of Self-Healing: A Practical Guide* – Vasant Lad
6. *The Tapping Solution* – Nick Ortner
7. *The Circadian Code* – Dr Satchin Panda
8. *Last Chance to See* – Douglas Adams
9. *Tuesdays with Morrie* – Mitch Albom
10. *On a Wing and a Prayer: Spirituality for the Reluctant, the Curious and the Seeker* – Kushal Choksi
11. *The Golf Stories* – P.G. Wodehouse
12. *The Blandings Castle Stories* – P.G. Wodehouse

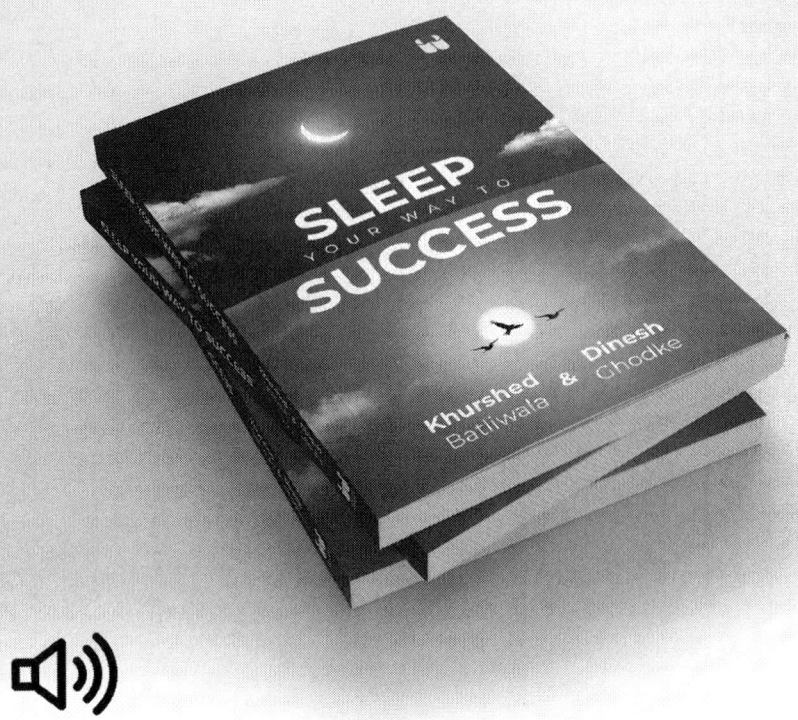

Sleep Your Way to Success - The Audio Book

Enjoy listening to Sleep Your Way to Success as an audio book. Narrated by the authors themselves, and packed with extra goodies, this is an incredible resource for everyone.

Here's what you'll get:

- The Entire Book – Sleep Your Way to Success
- Guided Meditations with Dinesh and Khurshed
- Soothing bed time chants
- Bonus chapters on The Biggest Obstacle to Success and Being Moneywise
- Recordings of QnA Sessions that Khurshed and Dinesh have conducted around the subjects of Sleep and Success
- More than 8 hours of content
- Other downloadable goodies

This audio book is available exclusively from our website
www.booksbybnd.com/sys/audiobook

Printed in Great Britain
by Amazon